WOMEN
and
AGING

Recent Titles in
Bibliographies and Indexes in Gerontology

Retirement: An Annotated Bibliography
John J. Miletich, compiler

Suicide and the Elderly: An Annotated Bibliography and Review
Nancy J. Osgood and John L. McIntosh, compilers

Human Longevity from Antiquity to the Modern Lab: A Selected,
Annotated Bibliography
William G. Bailey, compiler

Federal Public Policy on Aging since 1960:
An Annotated Bibliography
William E. Oriol, compiler

European American Elderly:
An Annotated Bibliography
David Guttmann, compiler

Legal Aspects of Health Care for the Elderly: An Annotated Bibliography
Marshall B. Kapp, compiler

Crime and the Elderly: An Annotated Bibliography
Ron H. Aday, compiler

Jewish Elderly in the English-Speaking Countries
David Guttmann, compiler

WOMEN
and
AGING

A Selected, Annotated Bibliography

Compiled by
Jean M. Coyle

Bibliographies and Indexes in Gerontology, Number 9
Erdman B. Palmore, Series Adviser

GREENWOOD PRESS
New York • Westport, Connecticut • London

Library of Congress Cataloging-in-Publication Data

Coyle, Jean M.
  Women and aging : a selected, annotated bibliography / compiled by
Jean M. Coyle.
    p.   cm. — (Bibliographies and indexes in gerontology, ISSN
0743-7560 ; no. 9)
  Includes indexes.
  ISBN 0-313-26021-4 (lib. bdg. : alk. paper)
  1. Aged women—United States—Bibliography. 2. Middle aged women—
United States—Bibliography. I. Title. II. Series.
Z7164.O4C68   1989
[HQ1064.U5]
016.3052'6'0973—dc 19   88-28975

British Library Cataloguing in Publication Data is available.

Library of Congress Catalog Card Number: 88-28975
ISBN: 0-313-26021-4
ISSN: 0743-7560

First published in 1989

Greenwood Press, Inc.
88 Post Road West, Westport, Connecticut 06881

Printed in the United States of America

The paper used in this book complies with the
Permanent Paper Standard issued by the National
Information Standards Organization (Z39.48-1984).

10 9 8 7 6 5 4 3 2 1

Z
7164
.O4
C68
1989

Dedicated to my mother, Bertha Jeanette Lay Coyle,
and to my early teacher, Elizabeth VonderOhe Brown

Contents

Series Foreword by Erdman B. Palmore   ix

Preface   xi

Acknowledgments   xiii

Introduction   xv

Roles and Relationships   1

Economics   21

Employment   29

Retirement   37

Health   43

Sexuality   59

Religion   63

Housing   67

Racial and Ethnic Groups   73

Policy Issues   87

International Concerns   91

Middle Age   99

General   103

Appendix   123

Subject Index   125

Author Index   129

Series Foreword

The annotated bibliographies in the Bibliography and Indexes in Gerontology series provide insight to the question, "What is known in the field of gerontology?" The purpose is simple, yet profound: to provide comprehensive reviews and references of the work done in various fields of gerontology. Since it is no longer possible for professionals to explore the vast body of research and writing in a subspecialty without years of work, annotated bibliographies are invaluable tools to the researcher.

This fact has become true only in recent years. When I was an undergraduate at Duke (class of '52), I doubt anyone had even heard of gerontology. Almost no one was identified as a gerontologist. Now there are over 5,000 professional members of the Gerontological Society of America. When I was an undergraduate, there were no courses in gerontology. Now there are thousands of courses offered by most major (and many smaller) colleges and universities. When I was an undergraduate, there was only one gerontological journal, **The Journal of Gerontology,** first published in 1945. Now there are over forty professional journals and several dozen books in gerontology published every year.

The reasons for the dramatic growth in gerontological interest are clear: the dramatic increase in the number of aged; the shift from family to public responsibility for the security and care of the elderly; the recognition of aging as a social problem; and the growth of science in general. The explosive growth in knowledge in this field has resulted in the need for new solutions to the old problem of comprehending and "keeping up" with a field of knowledge. The old indexes and library card catalogues have become increasingly inadequate for the job; they are cumbersome and unwieldy to use, and keeping them current is an arduous task. On-line computer indexes and abstracts are one solution, but make no evaluative selections nor organize sources logically as is done here. Annotated bibliographies are also more widely available than on-line computer indexes.

These bibliographies are useful to researchers who need to know what research has (or has not) been done in their field. The annotations contain enough information so the researcher usually does not have to search out the original articles. In the past, review of literature has often been haphazard and rarely comprehensive because of the large investment of time (and money) that would be required for a truly comprehensive review. Now, using these bibliographies, researchers can be more confident that they are not missing important previous research, duplicating past efforts or reinventing the wheel. It may well become standard and expected practice for researchers to consult such bibliographies even before they start their research.

Women are the largest and certainly one of the most important groups among the elderly. Even though much more research is needed on them, the literature is already vast, as shown by the 622 entries in this bibliography. Research in this field is becoming ever more important as the number of elderly women continues to increase faster than the number of men. As the literature demonstrates, most elderly women are rather different from most elderly men in many ways: problems, resources, abilities, opportunities, health, and longevity. This is the result of biological, psychological, social, and cultural differences between the sexes. It is usually not sufficient to talk about the elderly without recognizing the important differences between men and women.

This book is needed not only by academicians and researchers, but also by the practitioners who work with the aged, by older women, and by anyone who wants better to understand elderly women.

The author of this bibliography has done an outstanding job of covering all the relevant literature and organizing it into easily accessible form. Not only are there 622 annotated references organized into thirteen sections, but there are also an author index and a comprehensive subject index with many cross-references for the items in the bibliography. Thus, one can look for relevant material in this volume in several ways: (1) look up a given subject in the subject index; (2) look up a given author in the author index; (3) turn to the section that covers the topic; or (4) look over the introduction for a basic orientation to the field.

Dr. Jean Coyle is an unusually qualified expert in the area of elderly women because she has done considerable research in the field. Furthermore, she has provided expert consultation on several national programs dealing with older women and has taught at universities in Indiana, Texas, Louisiana, Illinois, Washington, D.C., and Virginia. Her annotations are concise and clear and one can easily understand the essence of the reference and determine whether the original is worth pursuing.

So, it is with great pleasure that we add this bibliography to our series. We believe you will find this volume to be the most useful, comprehensive, and easily accessible reference work in its field. I would appreciate any comments you may care to send me.

Erdman B. Palmore
Center for the Study of Aging and Human Development
Box 3003, Duke University Medical Center
Durham, NC 27710

Preface

This book is designed to provide an extensive selected bibliography on the topic of women and the aging process. While the primary focus is on the older woman, references also are included on middle-aged women. Both pragmatic and theoretical references are included.

Over 600 annotations are included. On some topics, very few references were discovered, which certainly would seem to indicate areas where research is needed. All references, with a very few exceptions, were published from 1980 through early 1988. Thus, very current information is being provided to the reader.

These annotated references are meant to serve as guides to relevant materials on women and aging. While research results are reported in some annotations, the primary objective was to give the reader extensive references to useful and appropriate documents, rather than to attempt to report "the whole story" in each case or to critique the documents.

Within each chapter, annotations are divided into books, articles, films, government documents, and dissertations. All materials identified are accessible through basic library systems.

The major areas covered herein include roles and relationships, economics, employment, retirement, health, sexuality, religion, housing, racial and ethnic groups, policy issues, international concerns, and middle age. Also included is an extensive selection of general items which did not fit neatly into any of the aforementioned categories. The subjects were perceived by the author to be basic and important areas of concern and interest with regard to mid-life and older women.

Acknowledgments

I would like to acknowledge the assistance of Erdman Palmore, series editor, and Mary Sive and Loomis Mayer, past and present editors, behavioral and social sciences, Greenwood Press, for their support in the development of this bibliography.

Able and thoughtful assistance in identifying relevant materials for this manuscript was provided by staff members in several divisions of the Library of Congress, The National Council on the Aging Library, and the Resource Center of the American Association of Retired Persons, all located in Washington, D.C.

I have appreciated very much, for over 30 years, the encouragement of my fifth grade teacher, Elizabeth Brown, in my diverse professional activities. Early writing lessons I learned from author Vardine Moore and English teacher Mary Alana Lahr, and early love of reading and writing from the many, many librarians I have known.

I am very grateful for the counsel and instruction provided by friend and colleague Sara Rix in the computerization of this manuscript--her patience and advice were much appreciated.

Finally, there are so many different role models of middle-aged and older women which have been provided in my life--Ruth Layfield-Faux, Louise Parsons, Kay Wood, Millie Seltzer, Heather McKenzie, Eulalee Anderson, Gertrude Leich, Dorothy Kreipke, Anne McCarrick, Juanita Daniels, Elizabeth Dean, Marie Fuller, Helen Ferguson, and Levenia Hunter are but a few.

Introduction

The study of aging elicits a focus on the study of women. During the last two decades, the older population grew more than twice as fast as the rest of the population (U.S. Senate, 1). In 1986, among persons 65 years old and over, there were 17.4 million women and 11.8 million men (U.S. Senate, 20). Within that older populace, elderly women outnumber elderly men three to two (U.S. Senate, 20). Among individuals 85 and over, there are only 40 men for every 100 women (U.S. Senate, 1). Statistically, the average woman lives longer than the average man, and, thus, is more likely to end up living alone (U.S. Senate, 20). Accordingly, older women, in general, experience longer retirement periods than do older men (U.S. Senate, 20).

Sex and race are important factors in determining life expectancy, but sex has now become the dominant factor over race (U.S. Senate, 25). The racial hierarchy in life expectancy shows white females to have the highest life expectancy at birth, followed by black females, white males, then black males (U.S. Senate, 27). Life expectancy at age 65 is increasing rapidly (U.S. Senate, 25). Between 1900 and 1985 elderly men gained 3.1 years and older women 6.4 years (U.S. Senate, 25). Bureau of the Census data (Spencer, 1984) project an additional 2.8 years for older men by 2050 and a gain of 4.5 years for older women.

Given these demographic data supporting the proportional representation of women in the total U.S. population, "it is ironic...that older women have been discovered so lately by gerontologists and the general public" (Markson, 1983).

While women have been the subject of much scholarly and popular attention within the last decade, only recently has research focused specifically on older women and the ways in which their aging processes may be similar [to] or distinct from those of men. It was not until 1978 [italics added] that the Baltimore Longitudinal Study added women to its study of normal aging; it was also in 1978 that the Annual Meeting of the Gerontological Society of America first placed a significant emphasis on older women (Markson, 1).

Sociologist Alice Rossi noted, in 1985, that she encouraged the view that "theories on sex and gender are not adequate if they are limited to social, economic, and political constructs. To examine gender in a life span framework encourages an awareness that our theories must embrace biopsychological constructs as well" (Rossi, XIII).   Rossi further cited the view that

> theories of aging are not adequate without a specification of gender...Gender often went unnoted in research at the two ends of the human life span...Research instruments in social gerontology typically inquire about relations with parents,... rather than in gender-specific terms, with mothers...Yet we know that across most of the life span from childhood to late middle age, social relations are structured in important ways along gender lines. To "neuter" premature infants and elderly persons seemed very strange indeed (Rossi, XIII).

While social scientific data on older women are limited, often, to extrapolation from statistics, "data focusing on middle-aged women, the future majority within the minority, are virtually nonexistent. It is only during the past decade that publications on the subject of middle-aged women in the United States have begun to appear in significant numbers, indicating that their authors are pioneering a new and important field of study" (Borenstein, 39). Until recent years, the study of mid-life focused on men (Baruch and Brooks-Gunn, 6). Baruch and Brooks-Gunn suggest that mid-life women may not share the same sense of imminent mortality or of inadequate accomplishment in the world as mid-life men, indicating that "the large differential in life expectancy between males and females...may well influence the intensity of such concerns" (Baruch and Brooks-Gunn, 6).

> For those mid-life women who were young adults in the 1940s and 1950s, an era when, far from being held to unattainable standards of professional accomplishment, achievement outside the role of wife and mother was unexpected, almost forbidden, the female version of "too short a time left, too much to do" is often "I have almost too many years left, and the chance to fill them with more than I ever thought I could" (Baruch and Brooks-Gunn, 6).

Another research bias affecting the images of mid-life women is the undue attention given to menopause and "the empty nest," while these predictable occurrences "rarely prove burdensome" (Baruch and Brooks-Gunn, 7).

> New ideas and opportunities...have changed the nature of the realities women face as they grow older, and mostly in a positive direction...The feeling that one's life is over after 40--that the primary task as mother is done and the best years past-- seems less and less widespread among today's midlife women. New educational and occupational opportunities, although far from adequate, are transforming the midlife experience for many women (Baruch and Brooks-Gunn, 7-8).

The "double standard of aging," explained by Susan Sontag as combined sexism and ageism, is readily apparent when contrasting demographic statistics and the remaining paucity of gender-specific gerontological literature. Identification of the gender of subjects, as has been noted, is not a given in research reports. For images to change, for the "double standard" to disappear, increasing scientific data are needed.

As Sontag indicated, over a decade ago, while both men and women may be penalized by becoming older, women are penalized much more severely than are men (Sontag). As Sontag notes, while men are viewed as moving from youthful good looks to the craggy, gray-haired distinguished nature of maturity, the basic standard of physical attractiveness for American women is "youthful beauty--unlined and ungray" (Sontag).

With the obvious, increasing physical changes of age for women, it may be difficult for even the most self-assured woman, as she grows older, not to harbor some doubts not only about her physical attractiveness, but also about her basic competence in dealing with life.   After all, the identifiably "masculine" traits such as "competence, autonomy, and self-control" are likely to increase with age and experience, while the "feminine" characteristics of being "helpless, passive, and non-competitive" do not improve with age (Sontag).   Women, of course, have acquiesced in this double standard, this system of inequality, and, thus, have helped to perpetuate it (Sontag).

Society's image of the older woman, as well as her own self-image, often presents the older woman as socially devalued, sick, sexless, uninvolved, and alone (Payne and Whittington).   The sparse scientific data which exist actually show no significant difference between older males and females in health and functioning (Payne and Whittington); life expectancy rates, for one thing, would corroborate this.   Women alone in their later years have been found to complain of loneliness, but also to confess enjoyment with their new-found freedom and independence (Payne and Whittington).   The image of grandma in the rocking chair, while still widely accepted, is not always true.

The picture drawn by Sontag, then, shows older women in America as being stereotyped, doubly victimized by sex and age, and, often, not in an enviable economic position.   However, the depiction herein also allows for changing public and self-images and for individual and group potential in moving beyond the stereotypes to create more positive images, roles, and economic situations.

Since women represent a sizeable majority of the aging population, all issues of aging are intrinsically connected with women's issues.   However, whatever the topic, examination must be made of the special impact which these issues may have on women. Are women affected at an earlier age than men by certain situations?   Are assumptions made about men and women playing traditional roles?   Is women's longevity a factor in the situation?   How does sexism affect the problem?

> The aging establishment must come to grips with the fact that women alone are by far the largest constituency in all aging programs.   Policies should be determined with recognition that the major problems of aging--poverty, loneliness,   vulnerability   to   crime   and   to   institutionalization--are overwhelmingly the problems of unmarried women...As older women increase in numbers and become more active in their own behalf, they will gain in political and social clout.   Increasing numbers of older women will tend to give this segment of the population greater visibility, and increased involvement will add to our legitimacy as a group in society...The potential for older women to effect changes in our own lives, as well as in the social fabric, is growing rapidly...Older women must work to be included in policy making and leadership roles, especially in programs in which we are the primary constituents (MacLean).

Preparation of this manuscript provided ample evidence, early on, of the increase in interest in research on various issues affecting women as they age, even from 1980 forward.   In most areas included in this book, the difficulty lay not in finding relevant material but rather in selecting the most appropriate items for inclusion.   Some areas seem still to be lacking in research efforts or even to include gender as a stated variable, but the quantity and quality of research on women and the aging process are increasing.

Some of the topics covered in these chapters have been the foci of more research than have others.   There are numerous publications about widowhood and menopause, as examples; far fewer about middle-aged and older women and religious issues or policy issues.   For the researcher interested in issues affecting middle-aged and older women, the opportunities for research still are abundant.   Much more current research needs to identify gender as a variable in reporting research results.   In addition, gerontological and other researchers need to recognize the importance of investigating, especially in longitudinal studies, the behavior patterns, attitudes, and causative variables in women's lives. Given the considerably higher percentages of women than men in each succeeding age cohort, the gaps which still exist in valid information about women's aging patterns should dismay the serious researcher, indeed, the scientific community.

A survey of the literature reviewed in this manuscript reveals not only, however, the gaping holes which exist today, but also the amount of gerontological literature developed primarily in the past decade which <u>has</u> included gender as a variable or which has emphasized concerns of women.

Roles and relationships

The multiple roles and diverse relationships of many women may create complex life patterns. A "displaced homemaker," for instance, may need to re-enter the labor force after experiencing divorce or widowhood and find that her job skills must be updated, that she must learn new jobsearch techniques, that she is entering a technologically-advanced labor force.

Adjusting to widowhood is a typical experience of later life for the average American woman. Increasingly, more women must adapt to being divorced at mid-life or later. Multi-generational families--and the concordant role-playing--are becoming more common. Playing the role of an adult child with one's aging parents requires adaptation. Older women/younger men relationships still face powerful societal taboos. What becomes the life situation for the older "ever single" woman?

Economics

Older individuals have "substantially less cash income than those under 65" (U.S. Senate, 2) and are more likely than other adults to be poor (U.S. Senate, 1). Older women of every marital status (in 1986) had low personal incomes (U.S. Senate, 47). In every age group, older women were "substantially more likely to be poor than [were] men of the same age" (U.S. Senate, 47). In 1986, the median income of older females was 56 percent the median income of older males--$6,425 compared to $11,544 (U.S. Senate, 2). Almost three-fourths of the elderly poor are women (U.S. Senate, 2).

With regard to marital status, elderly women living alone had a more precarious economic status due to lack of financial support [from spouses] than did married women (U.S. Senate, 47). Married women had the lowest median income because they continued to depend on a spouse's income, but also were likely to benefit from a spouse's income (U.S. Senate, 47).

Bringing Social Security provisions into congruence with the contemporary roles of women is important, as is continued examination of the effects of work history and early family roles on prospective economic status at retirement.

Employment and retirement

Often due to great financial need, older women may continue, or start, working, in order to support themselves and their families. The "displaced homemaker," who has lost her "dependent" homemaker role through divorce or widowhood, may be very unprepared to move into the labor force, although she may be very needy in an economic sense. Women workers are disproportionately represented in the full-time, low-income work force (McEaddy, 17-24).

Employment and retirement remain closely-related issues for midlife and older women. Re-entry into the labor force, career continuation, or career change constitute issues of concern for women as they age. Increased labor force participation of women has direct implications for older women in the future (Marshall). Women as permanent and integral parts of the labor force must be recognized (Marshall). Block's 1982 study revealed that significant factors of satisfaction with retirement were not subjects' work patterns nor their social resources, but rather were health, preretirement planning, and income after retirement.

When the author was completing a doctoral dissertation on Job Involvement, Work Satisfaction, and Attitudes Toward Retirement of Business and Professional Women in 1976, it was difficult to locate relevant literature sources. Despite the participation of millions of American women in the labor force for decades, little attention has yet been paid to their planning for a retirement exit from that labor force. An emphasis on research on gender differences in preretirement planning and in the retirement transition is especially important (as George et al. note, 1984) because so many previous studies have included only men, the labor force participation rates among women have risen (with coincidental need for information about the retirement of these workers), and there is still limited evidence about sex differences in retirement and retirement preparation. Existing studies on female retirement are based on unrepresentative and/or small samples, with some contradictory results (Szinovacz). In 1976 there was a dearth of studies investigating the work and retirement attitudes of women, with most retirement studies (with the exception of researchers such as Streib and Schneider and Jaslow) being marked "by the total exclusion of females, by small, nonrepresentative samples of women, and/or by the omission of analysis by sex" (Coyle). Most of the available literature on retirement is still male-oriented.

Longitudinal research is critical, as is consideration of the heterogeneity of women, occupational variations, economic differences, minority group membership, advanced technology, gender differences (and similarities), role flexibility, worklife pattern, occupational segregation, and support mechanisms.

Women's increased participation in the labor force has been substantiated, but women's reactions to retirement are still poorly understood...The increasing number of working women, the changes in society's definition of sex-based roles, and the inconclusive results of some of the research justify the need for further studies of women at work and in retirement from work (Rotman, abstract).

Maximiliane Szinovacz (1982) provides an appropriate summary of concerns related to women's work and retirement patterns:

General assumptions concerning the frequency and importance of women's participation in the labor force have led to an overemphasis on male retirement and a one-sided approach to retirement adjustment. It is argued here that the increased labor force participation of women has rendered female retirement a socially significant phenomenon, and it is precisely those characteristics underlying the neglect of women's retirement in the literature (e.g., discontinuous work histories, the importance of the empty nest, and widowhood) that may contribute to women's demonstrated vulnerability to the retirement transition. Therefore, women's retirement would also seem to constitute a policy-relevant issue, and retirement programs need to be adjusted to serve the divergent needs of male and female retirees...Research is especially needed on the retirement experiences of self-employed professionals, small business and private service workers, and the rural population. Additional efforts should be made to investigate retirement effects on minorities, who are overrepresented among low-income occupations and thus particularly susceptible to the negative effects of loss of income at retirement (Szinovacz, 20-21).

Health

Older women are more likely than older men to have chronic illnesses which cause physical limitations, while older men are more likely to have acute, life-threatening illnesses. Women more commonly experience arthritis and osteoporosis and men coronary heart disease (U.S. Senate, 98).

Difficulty with personal care activities is found among a greater proportion of women than men 65 and over, perhaps reflecting the older average age of women in this group. Women also have greater difficulty with home management activities, again, perhaps, reflecting the older age distribution of women and the phenomenon of more older women than older men routinely performing home management tasks and, thus, at greater risk of experiencing health-related difficulties with them (Dawson).

Women are more likely than men to enter a nursing home. "Nursing home residents are disproportionately very old, female, and white" (U.S. Senate, 118). For persons at age 65, the lifetime risk of institutionalization is 52 percent for women and 30 percent for men (Cohen).

While references on menopause abound, there is still a need for references on health promotion issues for middle-aged and older women and on other health care issues.

Sexuality

Women's experience of being sexual in midlife depends on women's age cohort, marital status, and the measure of being sexual used in a given study (Luria and Meade). Other research indicates the sexuality of women is influenced by gender (the social-psychological dimension of sex status) and by aging. "It appears that patterns of sexual behavior and attitudes about sexuality are more variable among women than among men at all ages" (Turner and Adams). Women generally experience little serious loss of sexual capability because of age alone. "Public acceptance of sexuality in later life is gradually increasing" (National Institute on Aging).

Religion

Alston and Alston and Blazer and Palmore, in separate 1980 studies, found that today's older woman is more religiously active than men. Women are more frequent church attenders and more religious in attitudes. Among females, religious activity remained significantly higher than that for males over time, but declined gradually for both men and women over time.

Housing

Living environments for older women are varied, ranging from independent residences to age-segregated and age-integrated residences to single room occupancy hotels to nursing homes. Women are more likely than men in the same age cohorts to enter a nursing home. Nearly 84 percent of nursing home residents are without a spouse. Since women tend to outlive their spouses and since absence of a spouse (or other family member) to provide informal support is the most critical factor in the institutionalization of an older person, older women become prime candidates for nursing home residency.

Racial/ethnic groups

Gender-specific research on diverse racial and ethnic groups is very much needed. While there has been increased focus on Blacks and Hispanices, much more information is needed on Native American elders and on older Asian Americans and the various immigrant groups, and, especially, on female cohorts within these groups.

Policy

Policy options for altering the condition of older women on global issues, sex roles, the health care system, employment, retirement, and life planning need to be developed. Cahn's summary of papers on policy proposals for midlife women indicates the expert contributors are "unanimous in stressing the importance of building a solid foundation in the middle years." Crucial issues for discussion include midlife women's future, role changes, displaced homemakers, retirement planning, education and training, employment, family, poverty, pensions, mutual help, and age discrimination.

International concerns

Aging for women is relative to the developmental status of the country of residency and origin--in a third world nation, a woman may be old in her forties. Thus, international perspectives on mid-life and older women must take into account these differences in definitions of aging.

The topics covered in these chapters were selected to encompass major areas of concern with regard to middle-aged and older women. Remaining gaps in the literature are readily discernible. Opportunities for research activity remain. The challenge is to promote research efforts to fill those gaps and to encourage gender-specific reporting in all gerontological research.

As Block et al. (1978) have indicated, "Despite their greater numbers, women have not been the focus of most major [italics added] research efforts in gerontology. The majority of researchers in gerontology have been, and are, male, and so tend to focus on the aging process of males."

Significant questions remain to be asked regarding age discrimination and employment status of older women, pensions and other retirement benefits, religious activity and beliefs, health perceptions and objective health status (mental and physical), housing options, effects of racial and ethnic characteristics, sexual behavior and attitudes, international perspectives, midlife concerns, economic status, and evolving roles and relationships.

The fact that the aging population is largely female, and that each decade over 65 has a larger percentage of women, has not yet permeated our thinking on the subject, in part because of the commonality of the aging experience. We all grow old, suffer a diminution of our physical well-being, social status and self-image. In addition, the significance of female aging has been masked by the myth of elderly couples sharing their twilight years (Sommers, 3).

Interest in aging has positive, non-altruistic aspects as well. "A potential alliance exists with those in their middle years who recognize that the most immediate way to prepare for later life is by improving conditions for those already old. It takes a long time to bring about any significant change; those in the middle years of younger would reap most of the benefits from senior activism" (Sommers, 17).

The responses to these questions and issues will provide implications for research, for public policy and legislation, and for involvement and action.

As a personal experience, old age is as much a woman's concern as a man's--even more so, indeed, since women live longer. But when there is speculation upon the subject, it is considered primarily in terms of men. In the first place because it is they who express themselves in laws, books and legends, but even more because the struggle for power concerns only the stronger sex (deBeauvoir).

Aging, as a universal human condition, is an essential focus for research, for policy, and for action. Targeting special subgroups within the middle-aged and older population, such as women, can only enhance our knowledge and our understanding of the particular interests and concerns of middle-aged and older women. By improving our awareness of this portion of the older population, indeed, we increase our comprehension of the total aging populace and of the aging process itself.

References

Alston, L., & Alston, J. (1980). "Religion and the older women." In Fuller, M., & Martin, C. (Eds.), The older woman, pp. 262-278. Springfield, Illinois: Charles C Thomas, Publisher, 343p.

Baruch, G., & Brooks-Gunn, J. (Eds.). (1984). Women in midlife. New York: Plenum Press, 404p.

Blazer, D., & Palmore, E. (1980). "Religion and aging in a longitudinal panel." In Fuller, M., & Martin, C. (Eds.), The older woman, pp. 279-285. Springfield, Illinois: Charles C Thomas, Publisher, 343p.

Block, M. (1982). "Professional women: work pattern as a correlate of retirement satisfaction." In Szinovacz, M. (Ed.), Women's retirement: policy implications of recent research, pp. 183-194. Beverly Hills: Sage Publications, Inc., 271p.

Block, M., Davidson, J., & Grambs, J. (1981). Women over forty: visions and realities. New York: Springer Publishing Company, 157p.

Block, M. R., Davidson, J. L., Grambs, J. D., & Serock, K. E. (1978). Uncharted territory: issues and concerns of women over 40. College Park, Md.: University of Maryland Center on Aging, 274p.

Borenstein, A. (1983). Chimes of changes and hours: views of older women in twentieth-century America. Cranbury, New Jersey: Associated University Presses, Inc., 518p.

Cohen, M., Tell, E., & Wallack, S. (1986). "The lifetime risks and costs of nursing home use among the elderly." Medical Care, 24(12), 1161-1172.

Coyle, J. (1976). Job involvement, work satisfaction, and attitudes toward retirement of business and professional women. Unpublished doctoral dissertation, Texas Woman's University, 247p.

Dawson, D., Hendershot, G., & Fulton, J. (1987). "Aging in the eighties: functional limitations of individuals 65 and over." Advance Data, No. 133, National Center for Health Statistics.

deBeauvoir, S., translated by O'Brian, P. (1973). The coming of age. New York: Warner Paperback Library, 864p.

George, L., Fillenbaum, G., & Palmore, E.   (1984).   "Sex differences in the antecedents and consequences of retirement." The Journal of Gerontology, 39(3), 363-371.

Luria, Z., & Meade, R.   (1984).   "Sexuality and the middle-aged woman."   In Baruch, G., & Brooks-Gunn, J.   (Eds.), Women in midlife, pp. 371-397.   New York: Plenum Press, 404p.

McEaddy, B.   (1975).   "Women in the labor force: the later years."   Monthly Labor Review, 98(ll), 17-24.

MacLean, J.   (Ed.).   (1981).   Growing numbers, growing force.   Oakland, California: Older Women's League Educational Fund, 56p.

Markson, E.   (Ed.).   (1983).   Older women. Lexington, Massachusetts: Lexington Books/D.C. Heath and Company, 351p.

Marshall, R.   (1983).   Work and women in the 1980s: a perspective on basic trends affecting women's jobs and job opportunities.   Washington, D.C.:   Women's Research and Education Institute, 26p.

National Institute on Aging, National Institutes of Health, Public Health Service, U.S. Department of Health and Human Services.   (1981).   Age page: sexuality in later life, 1p.

Payne, B., & Whittington, F.   (1976).   "Older women: an examination of popular stereotypes and research evidence." Social Problems, 23, 488-504.

Rossi, A.   (Ed.).   (1985).   Gender and the life course.   New York: Aldine Publishing Company, 368p.

Rotman, A.   (1981).   Professional women in retirement.   Unpublished doctoral dissertation, University of Pittsburgh, 271p.

Sommers, T.   (1976).   Aging in America: implications for women.   Washington, D.C.: The National Council on the Aging, Inc., 17p.

Sontag, S.   (1972).   "The double standard of aging."   Saturday Review, September 23, 29-38.

Spencer, G., & the U.S. Bureau of the Census.   (1984).   "Projections of the population of the United States, by age, sex, and race: 1983 to 2080."   Current Population Reports Series, P-25, No. 952.

Szinovacz, M.   (Ed.).   (1982).   Women's retirement: policy implications of recent research. Beverly Hills: Sage Publications, Inc., 267p.

Turner, B., & Adams, C.   (1983).   "The sexuality of older women." In Markson, E. (Ed.), Older women, pp. 55-72. Lexington, Massachusetts: Lexington Books/D.C. Heath & Company, 351p.

U.S. Congress.   Senate.   Special Committee on Aging, in conjunction with the American Association of Retired Persons, the Federal Council on the Aging, and the U.S. Administration on Aging.   (1987-1988).   Aging America: trends and projections. Washington, D.C.: U.S. Department of Health and Human Services, 186p.

Roles and Relationships

Books

001   Bailey, C.   (1982).   <u>Beginning in the middle</u>.   London, New York:
       Quartet Books, 271p.

Explores changes during the middle years.   Women have more opportunity to make
changes in their lives than is possible for most men.

002   Baruch, G., Barnett, R., & Rivers, C.   (1983).   <u>Life prints: patterns of
       love and work for today's woman.</u>   New York: New American
       Library, 291p.

Chapter on mothers and daughters.   Women often see their older mothers as role models
for their own aging.   Mothers' experience of the aging process seems to have a strong
impact on their daughters.

003   Baruch, G. & Brooks-Gunn, J., (Eds.).   (1984).   <u>Women in midlife</u>.
       New York: Plenum Press, 404p.

Interdisciplinary perspectives on present ideas about midlife.   Challenges existing myths and
stereotypes.   Examines roles and relationships for women in midlife and enhancement of
well-being.   Explores diverse experiences within cultural, racial, and socioeconomic groups.

004   Bastida, E., (Ed.).   (1984).   <u>Older women: current issues and problems</u>.
       (<u>Convergence</u>, Vol. 2).   Kansas City, Kansas: Mid-America Congress
       on Aging, 136p.

Considers the societal changes impinging on older women's lives.   Comprehensive
description of social and economic conditions affecting the older woman.   Topics include

health, crime prevention, social services, personal growth, and older women in rural areas and small towns.

005   Brown, J. & Baldwin, C. (1986). A second start: a widow's guide to financial survival at a time of emotional crisis. New York: Simon and Schuster, 223p.

Practical information to help widows make informed decisions about their lives. Combines practical advice and emotional counseling. Includes "action checklist" at end of each chapter, other lists and guidelines, sample form letters to insurance companies and others.

006   Cauhape, E. (1983). Fresh starts: men and women after divorce. New York: Basic Books, Inc., Publishers, 338p.

A social psychologist examines the effects of divorce at mid-life. Primary finding is that divorced men and women can master their circumstances and take power over their lives.

007   Cohen, J., Coburn, K., & Pearlman, J. (1980). Hitting our stride. New York: Delacorte Press, 280p.

Interviews and mailed questionnaires from 841 women aged 29 to 72, with the focus primarily on women aged mid-thirties to mid-sixties. In general, the women liked being the ages they were, and felt that the benefits of being older outweighed the losses of no longer being young.

008   Cohler, B., & Grunebaum, H. (with the assistance of D. M. Robbins) (1981). Mothers, grandmothers, and daughters: personality and childcare in three-generation families. New York: John Wiley & Sons, 1981, 456p.

Uses interviews, observations of families, and personality measures to consider relationships between young adults and their middle-aged or older mothers.

009   Davison, J. (1980). The fall of a doll's house. New York: Holt, Rinehart, & Winston, 240p.

Discusses women's roles regarding various housing environments.

010   Derenski, A. & Landsberg, S. (1981). Age taboo: older women-younger men relationships. Boston: Little, Brown & Co., 262p.

Describes various aspects of the relationships between older women and younger men. Looks at powerful societal taboos against such relationships and emphasizes how successful emotional commitments can be developed in such older woman/younger man liaisons through role flexibility.

011   Gross, Z. (1985). **And you thought it was all over!: mothers and their adult children.** New York: St. Martin's/Marek, 308p.

Describes the mothering period after children have left home for school, work, or marriage--the "orbital" stage of mothering following children's launching into the world outside the home.

012   Lopata, H. (1979). **Women as widows: support systems.** New York: Elsevier, 485p.

The author focuses on Chicago widows, basing her conclusions on interviews done in 1970. Her theoretical perspective is the role of support systems in the lives of these women.

013   Matthews, S. (1979). **The social world of old women: management of self-identity.** Beverly Hills, California: Sage Publications, Inc., 192p.

Uses the identity-constructionist perspective to consider older women. Emphasizes the problems of older women, and includes ideas on solutions.

014   Macdonald, B., with Rich, C. (1983). **Look me in the eye: old women, aging, and ageism.** San Francisco: Spinsters, Ink, 115p.

Collection of essays by the co-authors dealing with older women's issues, including the authors' lesbianism, the process and the politics of aging from their personal narratives.

015   Scott-Maxwell, F. (1968). **The measure of my days.** New York: Penguin Books, Ltd., 150p.

A personal journal by a well-known woman writer who, late in her life, trained as an analytical psychologist under Carl Jung.

016   Segalla, R. (1982). **Departure from traditional roles: mid-life women break the daisy chains.** Ann Arbor, Michigan: UMI Research Press, 151p.

Study of college-educated women 35-45, and of the alternative life styles that traditional, married women choose, often after their early childrearing years. Examines how these women are currently structuring their lives.

017   Seskin, J. (1979). **Older women/younger men.** Garden City, New York: AnchorPress/Doubleday, 143p.

Survey, through questionnaires, tapes, personal interviews, and group dialogues of older women and younger men involved in relationships. Observations on the "double standard of aging." "...The increase of older woman/younger man relationships can be viewed as a reaction against past repressions, as well as a steppingstone to new redefinitions of the bases of sexual attractiveness and emotional maturation." Describes a type of relationship, what may be a new major sociosexual trend.

018   Sheehan, S. (1984). Kate Quinton's Days. Boston: Houghton Mifflin Co., 158p.

Account of an independent Irish woman who has the emotional and physical problems associated with illness and who finds she must depend on others in her later years. A widow, almost 80, she relates her use of a new home care program.

019   Silverman, P. (1986). Widow-to-widow. New York: Springer Publishing Co., 227p.

Perspective on bereavement as a transition period, the development and implementation of the mutual-help widow-to-widow project, and how the widow-to-widow program has helped women adjust to being widows and to being women alone.

020   Sloan, B. (1980). The best friend you'll ever have. New York: Crown Publishers, Inc., 218p.

The author's personal account of bringing his widowed mother to live with his family.

021   Strugnell, C. (1974). Adjustment to widowhood and some related problems: a selective and annotated bibliography. New York: Health Sciences Publishing Corporation, 201p.

A comprehensive literature review on mutual help programs for widows. It is divided into such sections as: bereavement, widowhood, loneliness, role of women, mutual help groups.

Articles

022   Adams, R. (1985-86). Emotional closeness and physical distance between friends: implications for elderly women living in age-segregated and age-integrated settings. International Journal of Aging and Human Development 22(1), 55-76.

Seventy in-depth interviews of senior, unmarried women. Positive relationships were found between emotional closeness and physical distance, duration and emotional closeness, and frequency of interaction and proximity. Age-segregated housing enhanced development of emotionally close, local friendships.

023   Adams, R. (1987). Patterns of network change: a longitudinal study of friendships of elderly women. The Gerontologist, 27(2), 222-227.

White, non-married, elderly, middle-class women were interviewed and observed twice over a period of years. Middle-aged friendship patterns changed--subjects had more new friends than they had friends who had been eliminated or lost, but the average subject saw friends less frequently than she had in the past, felt emotionally distant from more friends, lived close to more friends, and had a denser network of friends.

024   Adams, R. (1985). People would talk: normative barriers to cross-sex friendships for elderly women. **The Gerontologist**, 25(6), 605-611.

Interviews and observations of 70 non-married, white, elderly, middle-class women. Cross-sex friendship is defined as romance and some norms inhibit romance during old age, while other norms encourage rejection of potential mates who cannot meet traditional sex role demands. Thus, elderly women may lack male friends.

025   Arens, D. (1982-83). **Widowhood and well-being: an examination of sex differences within a causal model. International Journal of Aging and Human Development,** 15(1), 27-40.

National survey data from National Council on the Aging 1974 study. Data support an overall decline in well-being for widowed persons. For widowed women, low economic resources are key in lower levels of well-being.

026   Beckman, L., & Houser, R. (1982). **The consequences of childlessness on the social-psychological well-being of older women. The Journal of Gerontology,** 37(2), 243-250.

"Widowed childless older women had lower psychological well-being than did widowed mothers," while childlessness had no significant effects on well-being of married women. Among older women, factors positively associated with well-being were physical capacity, religiosity, quality of social interaction, and strength of social support.

027   Braito, R., & Anderson, D. (1983). **The ever-single elderly woman,** in Markson, E. (Ed.), **Older women,** pp. 195-225. Lexington, Massachusetts: Lexington Books/D.C. Heath & Co., 351p.

Ever-single older women represent a small, but increasing, portion of the entire population. The group includes the socially isolated and those who are socially connected (maintain confidants).

028   Brody, E., Johnsen, P., & Fulcomer, M. (1984). **What should adult children do for elderly parents? Opinions and preferences of three generations of women. The Journal of Gerontology,** 29(6), 736-746.

Three generations of women were surveyed on their opinions of appropriate filial behavior toward elderly parents and on their preferences for providers of services which they might need in old age. Women preferred adult children as providers of emotional support and financial management but not of income. The middle generation was least in favor of receiving financial support or instrumental help from children, preferring to have formal sources of assistance.

029   Brody, E. M., Johnsen, P., Fulcomer, M., & Lang, A.. (1983). **Women's changing roles and help to elderly parents: attitudes of three generations of women. The Journal of Gerontology,** 38(5), 597-607.

Data from three generations of women on effects of women's changing roles on attitudes toward responsibility for care of elderly adults. "The oldest generation was most receptive (and the youngest the least receptive) to formal services for elderly persons, but all three generations agreed that old people should be able to depend on adult children for help.

Values about family care of elderly adults have not eroded despite demographic and socioeconomic changes."

030   Chiriboga, D. (1982). Adaptation to marital separation in later and earlier life. The Journal of Gerontology, 37(1), 109-114.

Examination of psychosocial functioning of recently separated men and women aged from the twenties to the seventies. Older subjects showed more psychosocial distress than did the younger subjects. While both sexes were equally optimistic about the future, women exhibited more psychological symptoms, greater emotional tension, more personal disorganization, and more life dissatisfaction than did men.

031   Erdwins, C., Tyer, Z., & Mellinger, J. (1983). A comparison of sex role and related personality traits in young, middle-aged, and older women. International Journal of Aging and Human Development 17(2), 141-152.

Four age groups of females--18-22, 29-39, 40-45, 60-75, were included in this study. Women over 60 and homemakers in their forties and fifties were strongest in conventional feminine traits.

032   Fallo-Mitchell, L. & Ryff, C. (1982). Preferred timing of female life events. Research on Aging 4(2), 249-267.

Examination of cohort differences in the preferred timing of events in the female life cycle. Middle-aged or old-aged women preferred earlier ages for family life events and later ages for general life events than did young adult women.

033   Feinson, M. (1986). Aging widows and widowers: are there mental health differences? International Journal of Aging and Human Development 23(4), 241-255.

From behavioral or psychological studies, there is no support for the idea that aging widowers have more emotional problems adjusting to widowhood than do aging widows.

034   Ferraro, K. (1985-86). The effect of widowhood on the health status of older persons. International Journal of Aging and Human Development 21(1), 9-25.

Data from Bureau of the Census interviews within the Survey of Low-income Aged and Disabled. The result of widowhood is an immediate decrease in perceived health among older people. Women and the old-old are "health optimistic" compared to men and the old. This health optimism is not diminished by widowhood.

035   Ferraro, K., & Barresi, C. (1982). The impact of widowhood on the social relations of older persons. Research on Aging 4(2), 227-247.

Panel data from a national survey of the low-income aged used. One of the most important findings was general stability of the recently widowed in regard to family relations. But for people widowed more than four years, there were lower levels of social interaction in terms of family contact.

036   Gentry, M., & Shulman, A. (1985). Survey of sampling techniques in widowhood research, 1973-1983. The Journal of Gerontology, 40(5), 641-643.

Focus on use and reporting of sampling procedures found in research on widowhood. Thirty-three percent of the studies did not report the sampling procedures used and most investigators who did identify their sampling procedures did not indicate awareness of the limitations of generalizations of their results because of their sampling procedures.

037   Goldberg, G., Kantrow, R., Kremen, E., & Lauter, L. (1986). Spouseless, childless elderly women and their social supports. Social Work, 31, 104-112.

Older women without a spouse or a child lack two primary sources of social support for the elderly. However, most of the spouseless, childless women in this study "had developed substitute supports for the close kin they lacked."

038   Hagestad, G. (1987). Family. In Maddox, G. (Ed.), The encyclopedia of aging, pp. 247-249. New York: Springer Publishing Company, 890p.

Women are "the linchpin of family contact, the kin-keepers." Due to gender differences in life expectancy, a woman is generally the oldest member of a family lineage.

039   Hagestad, G. (1987). Parenting. In Maddox, G. (Ed.), The encyclopedia of aging, pp. 511-512. New York: Springer Publishing Company, 890p.

Women attach different meanings to parenthood than do men. Women are more likely to describe their relationships with children as "affectively close, especially with daughters," and more likely to have their children become their confidants. Both men and women report feeling closer to their mothers than they do to their fathers.

040   Hand, J. (1983). Shopping-bag women: aging deviants in the city. In Markson, E. (Ed.), Older women, pp. 155-177. Lexington, Massachusetts: Lexington Books/D. C. Heath & Co., 351p.

A shopping-bag woman is defined, here, as "a homeless vagrant who lives in urban public places and who carries her household with her in shopping bags." The term, here, refers only to "women who have been homeless for at least one year and who have developed a stable life-style in that situation."

041   Hess, B. (1987). Friendship. In Maddox, G. (Ed.), The encyclopedia of aging, pp. 263-264. New York: Springer Publishing Company, 890p.

Includes section on friendship and gender roles. Reports that, at all ages, women are more likely than men "to describe their friendships in terms of intimacy, self-disclosure, and emotional closeness" and that "women's skills in seeking out and maintaining intimate friendships serve important adaptive and life-extending functions in old age, similar to those afforded to older men by a spouse."

042   Hess, B., & Waring, J. (1983). Family relationships of older women: a women's issue. In Markson, E. (Ed.), Older women, pp. 227-251. Lexington, Massachusetts: Lexington Books/D. C. Heath & Co., 351p.

Discussion of family relationships of women in old age, including old-age dependency, familial resources, childless women, parent/child bonds, caregivers to the elderly, and social policies affecting family relationships.

043   Homan, S., Haddock, C., Winner, C., Coe, R., & Wolinsky, F. (1986). Widowhood, sex, labor force participation, and the use of physician services by elderly adults. The Journal of Gerontology, 4(6), 793-796.

Study of relationships of widowhood, sex, and labor force participation with the use of ambulatory physician services by elderly adults.

044   Hooyman, N. (1980). Mutual help organizations for rural older women. Educational Gerontology, 5(4), 429-447.

Describes problems and needs of rural older women, proposes the mutual help organization as an option for them to use in meeting their needs, explains development and evaluation of a mutual help model for rural older women, and indicates educational implications of this methodology for working with rural older persons.

045   Johnson, C. (1983). A cultural analysis of the grandmother. Research on Aging, 5(4), 547-567.

Analyzes role of the contemporary American grandmother.   Subjects keep uniform conceptions of the traditional grandmother, even though they've been adapted with their own middle-age norms.

046   Kohen, J. (1983). Old but not alone: informal social supports among the elderly by marital status and sex. The Gerontologist, 23(1), 57-63.

Among subjects aged 55 and over, the widowed elderly generally had an advantage over the married.   Sex differences were similar between married and widowed elderly persons. Women indicated more anchorage points for expanding their social roles than did men.

047   Long, J., & Porter, K. (1984). Multiple roles of midlife women: a case for new directions in theory, research, and policy. In Baruch, G., & Brooks-Gunn, J. (Eds.), Women in midlife, pp. 109-159. New York: Plenum Press, 404p.

Midlife represents an evolutionary period of the multiple careers and multiple roles which many women have.   Midlife may bring life transitions including changes or disruptions in family life, changes in labor force participation, and alterations in emphasis or priority among women's multiple roles.

048   Longino, C., & Lipman, A.   (1982).   The married, the formerly
      married and the never married: support system differentials of older
      women in planned retirement communities.   International Journal of
      Aging and Human Development, 15(4), 285-297.

Exploration of informal support given to older women, depending upon their marital status
and the presence of living children.   Women presently or formerly married received more
emotional, social, and instrumental support from their family members, but having living
children determined receipt of more emotional, social, and instrumental support from their
families.   The greatest informal support deficits, among the never married, were seen to be
resulting from the lack of children.

049   Lopata, A.   (1987).   Widowhood.   In Maddox, G. (Ed.), The
      encyclopedia of aging, pp. 693-696.   New York: Springer Publishing
      Company, 890p.

Modernization trends in society have resulted in numbers of women who live independently
in widowhood, without control of the patriarchal family, and self-sufficient economically.
"Men are dying at a younger age than women, resulting in a disproportionate number of
widowers...There is no social role of widows, as there is in some other societies, and the
identity can lead to a rather gender-segregated life for women in this marital status."

050   Lopata, H., & Barnewolt, D.   (1984).   The middle years: changes and
      variations in social-role commitments.   In Baruch, G., & Brooks-Gunn,
      J. (Eds.), Women in midlife, pp. 83-108.   New York: Plenum Press,
      404p.

A major difference found between 1956 and 1978 Chicago area women is the devaluation
of role of housewife.

051   Markides, K., Costley, D., & Rodriguez, L.   (1981).   Perceptions of
      intergenerational relations and psychological well-being among elderly
      Mexican-Americans: a causal model.   International Journal of Aging
      and Human Development, 13(1), 43-52.

Sample of 98 Mexican-Americans aged 60 or over, with 60 women included.   Although
women were included, gender was not reported as a variable in these data.   The addition of
intergenerational solidarity to health, socioeconomic status, and activity contributed
significantly to explaining life satisfaction, but did not play a significant intervening role
except between health and life satisfaction.

052   Markson, E.   (1987).   Marital status.   In Maddox, G. (Ed.), The
      encyclopedia of aging, pp. 420-421.   New York: Springer Publishing
      Company, 890p.

In the United States and other industrialized nations, "patterns of marital status in later life
vary dramatically by sex."   Many more older men [than older women] are married.

053   Montgomery, R.   (1987).   Marriage.   In Maddox, G. (Ed.), The
       encyclopedia of aging, pp. 421-423. New York: Springer Publishing
       Company, 890p.

There is "a substantial difference between the marriage patterns of older men and older
women." Mot men remain married throughout their lives. The "likelihood of a woman
being married decreases substantially with age."

054   O'Bryant, S.   (1985).   Neighbors' support of older widows who live
       alone in their own homes. The Gerontologist, 25(3), 305-310.

Comparison of widows with no children, with children living elsewhere, and with children
living in the same city. Childless widows did not receive higher levels of support,
although they had, apparently, greater need.

055   O'Rand, A.   (1987).   Sex roles.   In Maddox, G. (Ed.),   The
       encyclopedia of aging, pp. 604-606. New York: Springer Publishing
       Company, 890p.

At midlife, both males and females may "face a variety of losses and gains in
expectations...midlife roles are not narrowly limited, but highly variable."   Both
convergence and loss may occur in late middle age and old age. Role convergence means
that there are fewer differences in the social worlds of men and women.

056   O'Rand, A.   (1987).   Women: changing status. In Maddox, G. (Ed.),
       The encyclopedia of aging, pp. 697-699.   New York: Springer
       Publishing Company, 890p.

"The shapes of women's lives have changed over the course of the twentieth century, but
the relative status of women in late life has not." Changes in life expectancy, fertility,
marriage, work force participation, and economic opportunities have enabled women to
participate more as individuals in many spheres of life. However, most late-life women
still have high risk of widowhood, ill health, and/or poverty.

057   O'Rand, A. M., & Henretta, J. C. (1982). Women at middle age:
       developmental transitions. The Annals of The American Academy of
       Political and Social Science, 464, 57-64.

Midlife role transitions for women are diverse and depend upon earlier life events
connected with marriage, childbearing, and work.

058   Premo, T. (1984-1985). A blessing to our declining years: feminine
       response to filial duty in the New Republic. International Journal of
       Aging and Human Development, 20(1), 69-74.

Examination of the ties that bound adult daughters to their aged parents in the late 18th and
early 19th centuries. The contemporary dilemma of filial duty has a long history.

059   Roberto, K. A., & Scott, J. P. (1984-85). Friendship patterns among
       older   women.   International   Journal   of   Aging   and   Human
       Development, 19(1), 1-10.

White, middle-class, urban women, 65 or older, were studied. Older widows received more
help from their friends than did married older women.

060   Roebuck, J. (1983). Grandma as revolutionary: elderly women and
       some modern patterns of social change. International Journal of Aging
       and Human Development, 17(4), 249-266.

Despite the disadvantages they have faced, women in western nations have coped
successfully with problems of aging "during the past century and have responded positively
to great social and personal changes."

061   Scott, J., & Kivett, V. (1985). Differences in the morale of older, rural
       widows and widowers. International Journal of Aging and Human
       Development, 21(2), 121-136.

Effect of sex differences on the morale of older widowed individuals. Sex of subject didn't
affect morale, but perceived financial status and self-rated health had significant direct
effects. Neither sex was more disadvantaged than the other by widowhood.

062   Sedney, M. (1985-86). Growing more complex: conceptions of sex
       roles across adulthood. International Journal of Aging and Human
       Development, 22(1), 15-29.

Examines conceptions of femininity and masculinity in women who were college freshmen,
in their mid-twenties, mid-thirties, and mid-forties. Older women showed a more
articulated view of roles and put a greater emphasis on the biological element of their role
and were more likely to reject the idea of a general relationship between gender and
personality.

063   Thomas, J.   (1986).   Age and sex differences in perceptions of
       grandparenting. The Journal of Gerontology, 41(3), 417-423.

Relatively young grandparents expressed the greatest willingness to provide childrearing
advice. Grandmothers indicated relatively high levels of satisfaction with grandparenting,
regardless of their grandchildren's ages.

064   Thurnher, M. (1976). Midlife marriage: sex differences in evaluation
       and perspectives. International Journal of Aging and Human
       Development, 7(2), 129-135.

Three life stages--newlyweds, middle-aged parents, and individuals about to retire--are
represented in a sample of white, middle and lower-middle class individuals. Examines
subjects' perceptions of marital relations. Middle-aged subjects placed the greatest emphasis
on role performance. Middle-aged women were the least positive in evaluating their
marriages.

065   Traupmann, J., Eckels, E., & Hatfield, E.   Intimacy in older women's lives. (1982). The Gerontologist, 22(6), 493-498.

Included in this study were 106 married women, aged 50 to 82. Subjects' life satisfaction and psychological well-being were strongly related to their satisfaction with their intimate relationships.

066   Wentowski, G.   (1985).   Older women's perceptions of great-grandmotherhood: a research note. The Gerontologist, 25(6), 593-596.

An exploratory anthropological study of 19 older women's perceptions of great-grandmotherhood.   Great-grandmotherhood was significant for symbolic and emotional reasons (rather than social and instrumental).

Films

067   Brigham Young University (producer). (1977). The mailbox. Brigham Young University, KENTSU, 1977. (Film, also video).

An elderly woman waits each day to receive a letter from children. Film depicts the loneliness of older persons when family members do not communicate meaningfully with them.

068   Carrell, I. & O. (Producers). Mrs. Kay: her failing marriage. Pictura Films.

After a 26-year marriage, Mrs. Kay finds her husband loves someone else. The story is of a middle-aged wife and mother whose children and husband have all left home, leaving her behind.

069   Films Incorporated. (1972). Harold and Maude.

A troubled young man and an old woman have an affair. She gives him the strength and courage to face his life.

070   Gilbert, B. (Producer).   On golden pond.   ITC Films/IPC Films, 1985(?).
An 80-year-old man and his wife spend a "final" summer at Golden Pond. Ethel, the wife, is optimistic and supportive of her husband.

071   Ideas and images. (1980). Lila.

Documentary of Lila Bonner-Miller. At 80 years old, she is an active psychiatrist, church leader, and great grandmother.

072   Lorimar (Producer). (1976). The Widow.

Effects of sudden widowhood. Based on autiobiography by Lynn Caine.

073   Mass Media (Distributor). (1970). A yellow leaf.

An older woman sitting in her rocking chair muses on her life, which she feels "ended" when her husband died in World War II.

074   McGraw-Hill Films (Distributor). (1963). Three grandmothers.

Comparison and contrast of the roles and lives of three grandmothers--from Nigeria, Brazil, and Canada.

075   New Day Films (Distributor). (1974). Nana, Mom and me.

Portrayal of the filmmaker, her middle-aged mother, and her grandmother--investigation of three different female generations.

076   Owens, J. (Producer).   (1980).   What shall we do about mother?
        (Film, also video).

Experiences of two families deciding what to do about their aging parents.

077   Peabody, P. (Producer). (1980). The female line.

Documents three generations of women in one family--Mary Parkman Peabody, activist; Marietta Tree, businesswoman and former United Nations Ambassador; and Frances Fitzgerald, Pulitzer Price-winning author.

078   Pinsker, S. (Producer). (1975). See no evil.

Story of unmarried couple in their seventies who live in a senior citizen hotel. Bertha, almost blind, has become very resentful of her loss of independence.

079   Stewart, P. (Producer). (1977). Opening night.

Portrayal of aging actress who faces a mid-life identity crisis by using alcohol and sex.

080   Stuart, M. (Producer). (1981). Widows. (Film, also video).

Experiences and coping techniques of old and young widows.

081   Sun Life Assurance Company of Canada (Producer).   (1971).   For tomorrow...and tomorrow.

Describes the problems of, and solutions for, widows in the United States, England, and Canada.

082   Teleketics, Franciscan Communications Center (Producer).   (n.d.). Hello in there. TKF.

A lonely widow uses her imagination to escape the monotony of her life in a retirement home.

083   University of California, Division of Cinema-Television in association with the Journey's End Foundation and the Andrus Gerontology Center (Producer).   (1982).   Grieving: suddenly alone.   (Film, also video).

A middle-aged woman, Kate, adjusts to her husband's death, discovers her own personal strengths, joins a widows' support group.

084   Widowhood.   (1979).   (Video).

Case study of widowhood, with an honest analysis and willingness to share experiences by widow Mary Gallagher.

085   WTTW-TV (Producer).   (1978).   Grandmother and Leslie.   PEREN.

Depicts the intergenerational relationships of a grandmother and an infant.

086   Brody, E. M. (n.d., released 1987).   Women-in-the-middle: the mental health effects of parent care.   Women's Mental Health Occasional Paper Series, National Institute of Mental Health, U.S. Department of Health and Human Services, 40p.

Describes issues of "women-in-the-middle," women helping a disabled elderly relative. These women most often are in middle age and are caught in the middle by multiple responsibilities that compete for their time and energy.

087   Veterans Administration.   (1984).   The aging female veteran: follow-up analyses from the survey of aging veterans.   Office of Information, Management, and Statistics, Statistical Policy and Research Service Research Division, 8 p.

Data from mid-1983 study.   The potential exists for female veterans to become more extensive users of Veterans Administration medical care facilities than male veterans, especially for nursing home and domiciliary care.

088   Veterans Administration.   (1983).   The female veteran population.
Office of Reports and Statistics, Statistical Policy and Research Service
Research Division. Washington, D.C., 15p.

Data on the female veteran population from the 1980 census, the first time statistical data
were collected on the female veteran population.   As more female veterans age, their needs
will correspondingly increase.

Dissertations

089   Allen, K.   (1984).   A life course study of never-married and ever-
married elderly women from the 1910 birth cohort.   Unpublished
doctoral dissertation,, Syracuse University, 233p.

Edited life histories of 15 never-married older women and 15 widows.   Five life course
careers were examined: family, friendship, work, health, and residence.

090   Anderson, R.   (1982).   Mothers and daughters: their adult
relationship.   Unpublished doctoral dissertation, University of
Minnesota, 141p.

Focus on emotional differences between mothers and daughters, ego development
comparisons, and types of relationships.   Evidence of continued importance of mother-
daughter relationship into adulthood, for women at all ego levels.

091   Barr, F.   (1984).   Role transition of reentry women.   Unpublished
doctoral dissertation, The University of Tennessee, 178p.

Explores role transition of women pursuing a delayed education.   Looks at factors
associated with presence or absence of role strain resulting from role accumulation.

092   Brown, B.   (1982).   Married, academic women in mid-life transition.
Unpublished doctoral dissertation, Temple University, 199p.

Investigated whether married, academic women in mid-life transition followed the same
developmental patterns as the men in Levinson's 1978 study.   Subjects followed the same
developmental patterns as the men in Levinson's study.

093   Clary, F.   (1983).   Life satisfaction among elderly widowed women.
Unpublished doctoral dissertation, University of Minnesota, 300p.

A positive relationship was found between style of coping of older widows and the
percentage of older widows who say that they are "delighted" with their life as a whole.

094   De Lago, L. (1986). Women at mid-life: mothers at home, mothers at work. Unpublished doctoral dissertation, University of Pennsylvania, 180p.

Case study of differences and similarities, at mid-life, between mothers who stay at home and mothers who go to work; four women were in the final sample. Report on time spent in different roles.

095   De Guilio, R. (1984). Identity loss and reformulation in young, middle-aged, and older widowed women. Unpublished doctoral dissertation, The University of Connecticut, 266p.

Exploration of effects of spouse death upon the identity and adaptation of widowed women. Middle-aged widows seemed to experience a more troubled adaptation in widowhood than did young or older widows.

096   Doliva, L. (1982). The effect of sex and age on the relationship between androgyny and self esteem. Unpublished doctoral dissertation, University of California, Berkeley, 165p.

This investigation revealed age and sex differences in agency scores, sex differences in communion scores, and age differences in androgyny scores.

097   Finkelstein, L. (1986). Psychosocial development of mid-life women enrolled as college undergraduates. Unpublished doctoral dissertation, Boston University, 225p.

Description of interrelationships between women's growth at mid-life (38-45) and their undergraduate college experience. The women experienced dramatic changes, seeming to become different people.

098   Friday, P. (1985). Coping with widowhood: a study of urban and rural widows. Unpublished doctoral dissertation, The University of Wisconsin, Madison, 277p.

Eighty elderly women were interviewed. Four coping patterns found, in order of frequency of use (highest first), were: managing psychological tension, social support, maintaining family integrity, and self development and reliance. There were no major differences discovered between urban and rural widows.

099   Greenaway, K. (1984). A comparison of the relationship between body image and self-concept in middle aged and younger women. Unpublished doctoral dissertation, York University (Canada).

Exploration of predictors of positive self-concept in women and the relationship of body image to self-concept in particular. Interpersonal relationships and physical appearance were the strongest predictors of self-concept.

100   Hottenstein, E. (1986). **The female mid-life student: a case study of three mid-life women at the Luzerne County Community College (Pennsylvania).** Unpublished doctoral dissertation, University of Pennsylvania, 201p.

Mid-life female students returning to post-secondary education were determined to have familial, financial, and personal stresses not faced by the traditional-aged student.

101   Kaye, A. (1981). **An investigation of early adult and midlife structure for women living a traditional life pattern.** Unpublished doctoral dissertation, University of Pittsburgh, 183p.

Traditional women, in this study, were defined as women who were primarily home-centered and sustaining a full-time homemaker life pattern throughout their adult years. Seventeen generic life themes emerged in the lived-experiences of the eight subjects across the developmental phases.

102   Krach, M. (1985). **Rural adults' perceptions of filial responsibility for and affectional bonds with their aged parents.** Unpublished doctoral dissertation, The Ohio State University, 148p.

Perceived levels of filial responsibility of rural, adult children for their elderly parents were found to be significantly related to their perceived levels of affection for their parents. The mean level of filial responsibility and affection was lower for females than it was for males.

103   LaFont, P. (1986). **Family support factors associated with the self-esteem of mature women enrolled in selected Louisiana colleges and universities.** Unpublished doctoral dissertation, The Louisiana State University and Agricultural and Mechanical College, 154p.

Investigation of factors of family support associated with the self-esteem of women over the age of 35 enrolled in selected Louisiana colleges and universities. Those subjects who had support from their children tended to have higher self-esteem than those who had no support from their children.

104   Lieberman, D. (1984). **Age-group responses toward the young-adult, middle-aged, and elderly in Athens, Greece.** Unpublished doctoral dissertation, The University of Florida, 131p.

To elicit word-responses of 125 male and female Greek nationals from various socioeconomic neighborhoods toward individuals of particular age and gender. All subjects were most positive toward the "middle-aged" label, neutral toward the "young-adult" label, and least positive toward the "elderly" label.

105   Massey, V. (1983). Older women and younger men: the initiation
       narrative of the French Eighteenth Century. Unpublished doctoral
       dissertation, Columbia University, 224p.

Examines the relationship between older women and younger men in the initiation novel
of the French eighteenth century. Focus on older woman as seducer, subject rather than
passive object.

106   McCrory, A. (1984). The impact of caregiving on the marital need
       satisfaction of older wives with dependent husbands. Unpublished
       doctoral dissertation, The University of North Carolina at Greensboro,
       149p.

Influence of caregiving on the marital need satisfaction of older women caring for
dependent, functionally-impaired husbands at home. The marital status of these subjects is
"long-term marital limbo."

107   Moss, W. (1981). An assessment of self-esteem and perceived needs of
       widowed and divorced women. University of Kentucky, 149p.

Examines relationship between self-esteem and selected variables for a sample of divorced
and widowed women who had become displaced homemakers.

108   Replogle, M. (1984). Explorations into the life of a nonagenarian
       woman: a new study of aging. Unpublished doctoral dissertation, The
       Union for Experimenting Colleges and Universities, 168p.

Explores the life of a nonagenarian woman and presents a study prototype for single-case
studies.

109   Sanders, G. (1983). Life satisfaction of older couples: a family
       strengths perspective. Unpublished doctoral dissertation, University of
       Georgia, 89p.

Explores relationship between family interaction quality and life satisfaction of older
persons. Variation in life satisfaction for female subjects was best explained by their
perception of their health, family strengths, and job prestige. The family strengths score
was a stronger predictor of life satisfaction for females than for males.

110   Shabad, P. (1983). The interpersonal needs of middle-aged and older
       married couples. Unpublished doctoral dissertation, Washington
       University, 174p.

In this study, there were found no statistically significant differences between interpersonal
needs of middle-aged and older, married couples. Age differences in marital satisfaction
were not shown.

111   Scharlach, A.   (1985).   Filial relationships among women and their
        elderly   mothers.   Unpublished   doctoral   dissertation,   Stanford
        University, 137p.

Examines the strain experienced by an adult daughter and the potential interference caused
by that strain with the daughter's relationship with her aging mother. "Findings provide
support for the hypothesis that mother-daughter relationships in later life can be improved
when daughters are helped to resolve potentially conflictual personal expectations regarding
their responsibilities to their aging mothers."

112   Stueve, C.   (1985).   What's to be done about Mom and Dad?
        Daughters' relations with elderly parents.   Unpublished doctoral
        dissertation, University of California, Berkeley, 239p.

Daughters were more attentive when they lived near their parents and the parents were in
poor health. Full-time workers tended to see and to help their parents less often.

113   Waciega, L.   (1986).   Widowhood and womanhood in early America:
        the experience of women in Philadelphia and Chester counties, 1750-
        1850. Unpublished doctoral dissertation, Temple University, 332p.

Examines the position of, and opportunities for, women in the late colonial and early
national America through consideration of the experience of widows in southeastern
Pennsylvania. The female capability extends well beyond the "woman's sphere...It was the
cooperation of widow and children together...which shaped how families responded to the
loss of husband and father."

114   Walters, J.   (1983).   Life satisfaction among urban and rural elderly
        widows. Unpublished doctoral dissertation, Michigan State University,
        171p.

Study of interaction of urban and rural elderly widows with their environments. These
subjects were highly competent, independent, with high life satisfaction and morale scores
and a high level of closeness with their children.

115   Wambach, J.   (1983).   Widowhood as the interruption and
        reconstruction of temporal reality. Unpublished doctoral dissertation,
        Arizona State University, 301p.

Describes sociopsychological aspects of the widow experience and analyzes these aspects
from a phenomenological framework. The widow experience process was an interruption
and a reconstruction of everyday temporal reality.

116   Whisler, E.   (1982).   Women's perceptions of factors affecting the
        nature and attainment of their ambitions: a three-generational study.
        Unpublished doctoral dissertation, Indiana University, 194p.

Describes women's ambitions across three generations within the same families, presents a
model that describes intervening factors in the formation and attainment of women's
ambitions, and shows the direction and degree of influence the three generations had on
each other's ambitions within and between cohorts and within and between families.

117   Whitted, M. (1983). An exploratory study: life satisfaction of elderly widows. Unpublished doctoral dissertation, The University of Michigan, 199p.

High satisfaction widows are optimistic, have good self-esteem, have formed and continue to form good social relationships, and have at least one activity which is important to them. The low satisfaction widow is depressed, doesn't have a particular activity which she enjoys, and has low self-esteem.

118   Wilson, K. (1983). Causes and consequences of divorce in late life. Unpublished doctoral dissertation, Portland State University, 196p.

Individuals divorcing in late life generally were urban residents, had low occupational status, few assets, weak religious and kinship ties. In this study, the primary cause of divorce was a longstanding lack of emotional gratification aggravated by some type of precipitating event. Females were found to have more negative divorce experiences and to suffer greater negative consequences than do males.

Economics

Books

119   Dissinger, K. (1980). <u>Old, poor, alone, and happy: how to live nicely</u>
       <u>on nearly nothing.</u> Chicago: Nelson-Hall, 261p.

This book for the older, poor woman covers how to get "a lot of mileage out of a little
money, how to enjoy life on a little money, and how to cope with the many problems that
confront the aging poor." There is discussion of budgeting, housing, clothing, food,
dieting, exercise, travel, illness, and decorating.

120   Figart, D. (1988). <u>Economic status of women in the labor market and</u>
       <u>prospects for pay equity over the life cycle.</u> Washington, D.C.:
       American Association of Retired Persons, 46p.

Suggests policy options concerning women in the U.S. labor force. Reports projects that
"six of ten new entrants to the labor force will be women and will comprise an increasing
percentage of the labor force in older age groups." Projections such as these and the
declining economic position of women over the life cycle emphasize the need to develop
public policies focusing on the special problems of older women.

121   Rix, S., with the assistance of Stone, A. (1984). <u>Older women: the</u>
       <u>economics of aging.</u> Washington, D.C.: Women's Research and
       Education Institute, 29p.

Using 1980 census data, the author indicates that "the majority status of women among the
aging population implies that aging is a women's issue. However, in terms of the equitable
distribution of resources among the aging, facing old age and responding to its needs is a
major social issue." The author predicts a "possibly" brighter picture for older women of
the future.

Articles

122   Hess, B. (1987). Poverty. In Maddox, G. (Ed.), The encyclopedia of
       aging, pp. 530-532. New York: Springer Publishing Company, 890p.

For many women, poverty in old age continues the poverty of earlier life. Women who
have faced discrimination in education and employment will face lower retirement benefits
later. For most older women, who are dependents of men, poverty is not a common
problem, but may become so, once a spouse dies. "The older the woman, the more likely
she is to live in poverty."

123   Kahne, H. (1981). Women and social security: social policy adjusts to
       social change. International Journal of Aging and Human
       Development, 13(3), 195-208.

The article describes the Social Security program and the lack of congruence of its
provisions with contemporary social roles of women and analyzes the potential impact on
women's status of alternative proposals, such as homemaker benefits. Concludes that
"reform based on societal consensus could increase equity of treatment and adequacy of
benefits for women."

124   Morgan, L. (1986). The financial experience of widowed women:
       evidence from the LRHS. The Gerontologist, 16(6), 663-668.

Reports of 606 white widows from the Longitudinal Retirement History Survey show that
many subjects have experience in managing money, some had discussed financial survival
with their spouses, less than one-third had received financial counseling as widows. Most
subjects are poor; prior experience with handling money did not decrease risk of poverty.

125   Morgan, L. (1983). Intergenerational economic assistance to children:
       the case of widows and widowers. The Journal of Gerontology, 28(6),
       725-731.

This article focuses on whether loss of spouse influences intrafamilial financial assistance
and whether gender of the surviving parent influences this. Loss of spouse does not reduce
the probability of support to offspring. The widowed woman is not less likely to continue
to assist her children than the widowed man.

126   O'Rand, A., & Henretta, J. (1982). Midlife work history and
       retirement income. In Szinovacz, M. (Ed.), Women's retirement:
       policy implications of recent research, pp. 25-44. Beverly Hills: Sage
       Publications, 271p.

Retirement income is much influenced by discontinuous work throughout life, a late age at
first job, and industrial location. "For unmarried women, any one factor may be a very
serious disadvantage, since their average expected income is very low. For married
women, work histories can have a surprisingly large effect on the couple's retirement."

127   O'Rand, A., & Landerman, R. (1984). Women's and men's retirement
        income status: early family role effects. Research on Aging, 6(1), 25-
        44.

Examines the effects of work history and early family roles on prospective economic
(income) status at retirement. The Earnings Record and Longitudinal Retirement History
Study of the Social Security Administration are used. Sex differences are particularly
apparent when considering the intervening effects of assets (net worth) and estimated
retirement incomes from private and government pensions.

128   Tracy, M., & Ward, R. (1986). Trends in old-age pensions for women:
        benefit levels in ten nations, 1960-1980. The Gerontologist, 26(3), 286-
        291.

The authors analyze women's pensions' development compared to men's over a 20-year
period in industrialized nations. In five countries, women's pension benefits did not keep
pace with men's benefits.

129   Uhlenberg, P., & Salmon, M. (1986). Change in relative income of
        older women, 1960-1980. The Gerontologist, 26(2), 164-170.

Income data from 1960, 1970, and 1980 United States censuses of the population reveal
that more recent old age cohorts have higher income distribution and some decline in
inequality among older women over 20 years. The status of older women to middle-aged
women has not improved. As they enter old age, cohorts still experience large income
decreases.

130   Warlick, J. (1985). Why is poverty after 65 a woman's problem?
        The Journal of Gerontology, 40(6), 751-757.

Families with aged male and female heads are compared on the composition of family
income. "The inferior economic position of women is due to deficient market incomes and
dependence upon deceased husbands for private and public pensions.   Policies that
encourage work and insure adequate survivor benefits will raise the relative economic status
of these families."

Films

131   WNED-TV. (1977). Age is money blues. PBS. (Also video).

Laurie Shields and Tish Sommers explain the "Displaced Homemakers Bill," a [then]
proposed national self-help program for women who have been homemakers and are being
excluded from the job market by age discrimination or a lack of marketable skills.

132   Klodawsky, H., & Sky, L. (1984). All of our lives. Filmakers Library.

Describes the situations of many older women, left without pensions or financial security.

Documents

133   Block, M. (1983). Working paper 3: income maintenance concerns of older women. National Policy Center on Women and Aging, University of Maryland, 46p.

The paper covers the economic status of older women, sources of retirement income, and income maintenance policy, with some consideration of options in other countries.

134   Communication from The President of the United States transmitting a legislative proposal entitled the "Pension Equity Act of 1983." (1983). 24p.

This legislation would amend the Employment Retirement Income Security Act (ERISA) and the Internal Revenue Code to provide greater equity in the provision of retirement income for women.

135   Grad, S. (1984). Income of the population 55 and over, 1982. U.S. Department of Health, Education, and Welfare, Social Security Administration, office of Retirement and Survivors Insurance and Office of Policy, 99 p.

The emphasis is on major sources of income for Americans 55 and over and the amounts received from such sources. Units of analysis are aged units and aged persons.

136   Iams, H. (1986). The 1982 new beneficiary survey no. 10, employment of retired-worker women. U.S. Department of Health and Human Services, Social Security Administration, Office of Policy, Office of Research, Statistics, and International Policy, 13p.

The study examines employment rates of women about 18 to 30 months after they first receive Social Security retired-worker benefits. Data are the 1982 New Beneficiary Survey, a nationally representative sample of new cash beneficiaries selected from the Social Security Administration's Master Beneficiary Record. Factors influencing the above-average employment rates of these women include lack of pension benefits, employment of at least 20 years' duration in their longest-held job, and being unmarried.

137   Strate, J. (1982). Working paper #3 of the National Aging Policy Center on Income Maintenance: post-retirement benefit increases in state pension plans: the response to inflation in the 1970s. The Florence Heller Graduate School, Brandeis University, 79p.

This article examines cost-of-living adjustments during the 1970s and their effect on the purchasing power of pension benefits. One-third of pension plans studied included teachers only.

138   U.S. Congress. House. Select Committee on Aging. 98th Congress. (1984). The economics of aging: a need for pre-retirement planning, 104p.

The report includes examples of particular older women and their problems, as well as mention of the spousal IRA bill.

139   U.S. Congress. House. Select Committee on Aging. Subcommittee on retirement income and employment. 97th Congress. (1983). The impact of Reagan economics on aging women: Oregon, 65p.

This document examines Social Security and income maintenance, impact of health care cuts on older women, impact of budget cuts on community service programs for the elderly, and impact of the Reagan budget cuts on older women.

140   U.S. Congress. House. Subcommittee on Labor-management relations of the Committee on Education and Labor. 97th Congress. (1983). Legislative hearing on pension issues, 293p.

This testimony is on problems caused by the failure of some health insurance trusts (METs) to pay beneficiaries' claims. Working women typically receive little or nothing in pension benefits compared to their male counterparts. Pension laws work against women working inside the home because a widow or divorcee may be left with no pension rights.

141   U.S. Congress. House. Subcommittee on labor-management relations of the Committee on Education and Labor. 98th Congress. (1984). Pension equity for women, 229p.

The document examines the private pension reform bill, HR 2100, part of the Economic Equity Act, "an attempt to improve the odds that women, be they homemakers or women working outside the home, will enjoy an old age of financial security." The Bill reduces the age for pension plan participation, vesting credit, and benefits accrual from 25 to 21.

142   U.S. Congress. House. Select Committee on Aging. 98th Congress. (1983). Women's pension equity, 369p.

This report describes the impediments which jeopardize or deprive women of a financially secure retirement. The report includes discussion of a federal portable pension system.

143   U.S. Department of Health, Education, and Welfare, Social Security Administration. (1986). A woman's guide to Social Security, 15p.

This guide to Social Security provisions may be of particular interest to women, since it includes information on career interruption, divorce, and widowhood.

144   U.S. Congress. Senate. Committee on Finance. 97th Congress. (1983). Potential inequities affecting women, 3 parts: 265p., 548p., 28p.

The Retirement Equity Act of 1983 relates to equality of economic and tax opportunities for women and men under retirement plans. The Economic Equity Act of 1983 relates to tax and retirement matters, dependent care program, nondiscrimination in insurance, regulatory reform and gender neutrality, and child support enforcement.

145   U.S. Congress. Senate. Subcommittee on Social Security and Income
       Maintenance Programs of the Committee on Finance. 98th Congress.
       (1983). Women's career choice equity legislation, 47p.

This legislation, S. 960, would correct some economic inequities against women--an IRA
provision, two Social Security provisions and a provision to amend the Walsh-Healy Act,
and Contract Work Hours and Safety Standards Act to remove the daily overtime
restrictions placed on federal contractors in the private sector.

Dissertations

146   Clark, L. (1983). Financial adjustment and satisfaction with level of
       living: a cross sectional view of female pensioners. Unpublished
       doctoral dissertation, The Florida State University, 174p.

The standards that women hold for satisfaction with level of living, the financial
adjustments that women make in retirement, women's satisfaction/dissatisfaction with
financial adjustments made in level of living following retirement are the foci of this
study.

147   Porter, K. (1985). The scheduling of life course events, economic
       adaptations, and marital history: an analysis of economic survival
       after separation and divorce for a cohort of midlife women.
       Unpublished doctoral dissertation, Syracuse University, 219p.

Economic survival for women whose first marriages have ended in separation or divorce is
compared with that of women who have been continuously married.

148   Primas, M. (1984). Friendship intimacy, financial security, and morale
       among elderly women. Unpublished doctoral dissertation, University of
       Maryland, 173p.

One hundred and forty elderly women are analyzed, with income appearing to be the
strongest predictor of morale of three of four hypotheses tested.

149   Schofield, R. (1985). The private pension coverage of part-time
       workers. Unpublished doctoral dissertation, Brandeis University, 282p.

The majority of part-time workers are women, who are disadvantaged in retirement income.
Data are from the 1979 Survey of Pension Plan Coverage by Social Security Administration
and the U.S. Department of Labor. The rate of pension coverage for full-timers is five to
six times that of part-timers, 51% compared to 9%.

150   Schuchardt, J. (1985). Objective measures of elderly women's
       economic well-being. Unpublished doctoral dissertation, Iowa State
       University, 92p.

Data from the 1979 wave of the Social Security Administration's Longitudinal Retirement
History Survey are used. Labor force participation had a significant impact on economic

well-being in retirement.   There are positive relationships between current income and receipt of financial transfers.

151   Silver, M. (1982). Life review as a developmental process: themes of caring, mourning, and integrity in group and individual therapy with low-income elderly women. Unpublished doctoral dissertation, Harvard University, 261p.

Twenty low-income women, 65 to 85, participate in 12 twice-weekly life review sessions. In the life review of elderly women, their mourning and concern with caring can be heard.

Employment

Books

152   Azibo, M. (1980). <u>The mature woman's back-to-work book</u>. Chicago: Contemporary Books, 178p.

This presents a practical and organized plan for entering and re-entering the work world emphasizing problems faced by single, divorce, separated, widowed, and married homemakers. "One's attitude is as important to the successful job hunt as is practical know-how. Perhaps more so."

153   Brodey, J. (1983). <u>Mid-life careers</u>. Philadelphia: Bridgebrooks, 248p.

A personal and pragmatic perspective of mid-life and mid-life career search. This book includes many personal examples related to mid-life career change, jobsearch techniques and strategies, setting goals, and preparing for middle age.

154   Fredericks, S. (1981). <u>How grandma got a job--in the business jungle</u>. Great Neck, New York: Todd & Honeywell, 42p.

The author uses her own life experiences as a model to provide information on finding employment via: self-assessment, goal setting, resume development, job search, and interview techniques. The book is aimed at the woman who has not previously worked in the labor force.

155   Hunt, H. (1984). <u>Senior women</u>. West Nyack, New York: Parker Publishing Co., 205p.

Written "to help senior women find ways to supplement their Social Security checks or other pension income." Step-by-step procedures of projects. Ideas include starting a mail order business, teaching sewing, property management, and handcrafts.

156   Kreps, J. (1971). Sex in the marketplace: American women at work. Baltimore: The Johns Hopkins Press, 117p.

Reviews literature on women's labor force participation--"when women work, at what jobs, and under what arrangements." Implications from these data for women's retirement periods.

157   Marshall, R. (1983). Work and women in the 1980s: a perspective on basic trends affecting women's jobs and job opportunities. Washington, D.C.: Women's Research and Education Institute, 26p.

Increased labor force participation of women has direct implications for older women in the future. Recognition of women as permanent and integral parts of the labor force requires particular attention to certain needs of women at various life stages, such as health care needs of older women.

158   National Association of Office Workers. (1980). Vanished dreams: age discrimination and the older worker. Cleveland, Ohio: The Association, 31p.

This report is the result of a nationwide survey of older women workers, interviews with staff of the Equal Employment Opportunity Commission, statistical research, and consultation with a wide range of experts in the field of aging. It is designed to aid older women workers and their advocates, government officials and policy makers, and actuaries in improving the working conditions and retirement situation of older women.

159   Shaw, L. (Ed.). (1986). Midlife women at work: a 15-year perspective. Lexington: Lexington Books/D.C. Heath & Co., 142p.

Contributions on employment consequences of different fertility behaviors, mature women and authority in the workplace, returning to school, women's labor market reactions to personal (family) crises, early labor market withdrawal, factors affecting remarriage, plans and prospects for retirement.

160   Shaw, L. (1985). Older women at work. Washington, D.C.: Women's Research and Education Institute, 16p.

Poverty is more common for women than for men. Provides profile of older women workers today--their work experience, education, occupations, earnings, pension eligibility; causes of low earnings--interrupted work careers, race, sex, and age discrimination, health problems; provides policy implications.

161   Shaw, L. (1983). Unplanned careers: the working lives of middle-aged women. Lexington, Massachusetts: Lexington Books, 149p.

Based on ten years of interviews of nearly 4,000 women from the National Longitudinal Survey of the Work Experience of Mature Women, started in 1967 by the Center for Human Resource Research at The Ohio State University. Nationally representative sample of women 30 to 44. Some data on black women. Chapters on re-entry to labor force, sex-segregated occupations, women's attitudes toward their roles.

162   Women's Research and Education Institute. (1984). Gender at work:
        perspectives on occupational segregation and comparable worth.
        Washington, D.C.: Women's Research and Education Institute, 26p.

Description of sex segregation in the workplace provides implications for economic status
of older women in the future.

Articles/chapters

163   Block, M. (1982). Professional women: work pattern as a correlate of
        retirement satisfaction. In Szinovacz, M. (Ed.), Women's retirement:
        policy implications of recent research, pp. 183-194. Beverly Hills:
        Sage Publications, Inc., 271p.

Three factors which were significant predictors of satisfaction with retirement were health,
preretirement planning, and income after retirement. Neither subjects' work patterns nor
their social resources were significant predictors of satisfaction with retirement. Author
suggests development of retirement programs for working women which emphasize
decision-making and goal-setting skills and knowledge of financial issues.

164   Brody, E., Kleban, M., Johnsen, P., Hoffman, C., & Schoonover, C.
        (1987). Work status and parent care: a comparison of four groups of
        women. The Gerontologist, 27(2), 201-208.

Study of parent caregiving daughters. The conflicted workers and subjects who had quit
work had the most impaired mothers and more of them (than the two groups of
nonworkers) had had lifestyle disruptions and caregiving strain.

165   Cassidy, M. (1985). Role conflict in the postparental period: the
        effects of employment status on the marital satisfaction of women.
        Research on Aging, 7(3), 433-454.

"Only the prestige associated with wives' present or former occupations and the husbands'
present or former occupations have significant effects on marital satisfaction." Their
employment statuses have no effect on marital satisfaction.

166   Depner, C., & Berit, I. (1982). Employment status and social support:
        the experience of the mature woman." In Szinovacz, M. (Ed.),
        Women's retirement: policy implications of recent research, pp. 61-76.
        Beverly Hills: Sage Publications, Inc., 271p.

Authors investigated whether the social support resources of women are affected by their
labor force participation, and found that the social support of the retired woman is a
function of her age, gender, and her participation in the labor force in later life. Authors
suggest that service agencies advertise through organizations in which retired women are
very engaged.

167   Grow, J. (1984). Opportunities for women in employment and training. In Women, work, and age: policy challenge, p. 11. Ann Arbor: Institute of Gerontology, University of Michigan, 26p.

Issues covered include the need for women to be prepared, that knowledgeable women are needed in greater numbers on the Private Industry Councils (PICs) and other employment and training boards, that educational programs must include vocational training that does not stereotype women into low-income jobs, enrollment in training and employment programs should be encouraged by provision of some benefits during the transitional period, legislation to raise poverty level and minimum wage level crucial, state civil rights laws should be enforced, more day care centers and job training programs needed so that young women, especially pregnant teenagers, can be helped to avoid a life of welfare or minimum wage jobs, women need comparable pay for comparable work.

168   Iams, H. (1986). Employment of retired-worker women. Social Security Bulletin, 49(3), 5-13.

Focus on variables associated with employment of women after they've received their first social security retired-worker benefits. Unmarried women consistently are more likely than married women to be working.

169   Kahne, H. (1985-86). Not yet equal: employment experience of older women and older men. International Journal of Aging and Human Development, 22(1), 1-13.

Examines importance of market equality of older working women and considers ways in which women's employment-related experiences differs from that of men--labor force participation rates, occupational distribution, earnings, unemployment, poverty, and retirement income. For women: rising labor force activity, traditionally different (from men) occupations, lower earnings, unemployment rates lower for women (although some may opt out believing no work is available), greater poverty, less adequate retirement income.

170   Keating, N., & Jeffrey, B. (1983). Work careers of ever married and never married retired women. The Gerontologist, 23(4), 416-421.

Subjected retired non-professional careers--relationship between marital status and involvement in a work career. Marital status affected the form of the work career (i.e., gaps in work more likely for married women) but not the quality of the work career.

171   Morgan, L. (1984). Continuity and change in the labor force activity of recently widowed women. The Gerontologist, 24(5), 530-535.

Findings from the 1975 Longitudinal Retirement History Study on changes in working caused by widowhood. Problems in locating employment for those not employed. Women already working were as likely to decrease their employment involvement because of becoming widowed as they were to increase it.

172   Riddick, C. (1985). Life satisfaction for older female homemakers, retirees, and workers. Research on Aging, 7(3), 383-393.

"Employment status had a significant effect on older women's life satisfaction." Currently employed older female subjects had greater life satisfaction than did their cohorts who were homemakers or retirees. Income and health problems meaningfully affected the life satisfaction of all three groups.

173   Rosen, E. (1983). Beyond the sweatshop: older women in blue-collar jobs. In Markson, E. (Ed.), Older women, pp. 75-91. Lexington, Massachusetts: Lexington Books/D.C. Heath & Co., 351p.

Focus on work-life experiences of older female factory workers in New England. Discussion of the nature and quality of blue-collar women's work experience and the conjunction between aging and industrial transformations. "These blue-collar women need full-time, paid employment for much of their lives. Despite the increasing economic insecurity, today's unskilled production jobs continue to provide stable employment for many older women who need them."

Films

174   WMHT-TV, PBSV. (1977). Arvilla. Video, Beta, VHS.

Portrait of Arvilla Groesbeck, 63-year-old woman dairy farmer struggling to survive in a male-dominated occupation.

175   University of Minnesota. (1974). Life career patterns of women. Video, Career Development of Women Series.

Seven women in different life patterns, including a black married woman who is in a mid-career shift and a divorced, re-entry woman, mother of six.

176   New Day Films. (1976). Union maids.

Three women in their sixties discuss organizing of trade unions--personal accounts of sitdowns, hunger marches, etc.

177   Wershba, J. (1983). The captain is a lady. Carousel Film and Video.

Biographical sketch of U.S. Navy Captain Grace Murray Hopper, who pioneered the development of computers during World War II. She became the oldest uniformed officer on active duty in the U.S. Armed Forces.

Documents

178   Benokraitis, N.   (1981).   Employment patterns of displaced
       homemakers: an exploratory study.   Washington, D.C.:   U.S.
       Department of Health and Human Services, 112p.

An examination of job characteristics, job entry/re-entry processes and perceptions of
important job attributes of displaced homemakers. Provides implications about training
programs for displaced homemakers.

179   Davidson, J. (1983). Working paper 2: employment concerns of older
       women. National Policy Center on Women and Aging, University of
       Maryland, 78p.

Covers economic status, labor force participation of older women, women as workers,
employment needs and opportunities, and employment policy options.

180   U.S. Congress. Joint Economic Committee. 98th Congress. (1984).
       The role of older women in the work force. Washington, D.C.: U.S.
       Government Printing Office, 117p.

The employment and retirement problems women meet in their later years are often a direct
result of a lifetime of job segregation, wage discrimination, and the difficulties of balancing
work and family responsibilities. Discusses how ageism, sexism, and, for minority women,
racism, also work against the full and productive use of older women in the work force.
"Congress must recognize the social realities facing older women today when it considers
changes in education, job training, dependent care, and retirement income legislation."

181   U.S. Congress. Senate. Committee on Labor and Human Resources.
       98th Congress. (1984). Women in transition, 189p.

Problems of women in transition, who, because of death, divorce, or disability of a spouse
suddenly became family head and who have rusty job skills or no marketable skills, women
trying to get off welfare dependence. Discussion of training programs which might help.

Dissertations

182   Gellert, J. (1986). An evaluation of the effectiveness of two career/life
       development programs for re-entry women. Unpublished doctoral
       dissertation, State University of New York-Albany, 118p.

Study of women over 24 who have not attended an educational institution or worked full-
time outside the home for at least three years prior to their attendance at these workshops.
"An intervention which specifically addresses teaching an awareness of the system and
strategies to enlist its support, increasing an internal locus of control, and applying
objective criteria to evaluation, and providing follow-up evaluation procedures is
significantly more effective in producing behavior change in locus of control, goal
attainment, and dyadic adjustment than one which is more general in its aims and
activities."

183   Gibeau, J. (1986). **Breadwinners and caregivers: working patterns of women working full-time and caring for dependent elderly family members.** Unpublished doctoral dissertation, Brandeis University, 313p.

Examines how working women manage their work lives while serving as primary caregivers for dependent elderly family members. "Working caregivers have significant, longstanding, and competing attachments to both their elderly family members and their employment."

184   Gordon, E. (1985). **The relationship of work to attitude toward retirement: a study of women in late middle age.** Unpublished doctoral dissertation, University of Pittsburgh, 227p.

The 1985 study explores the relationships between attitude toward work and attitude toward retirement among mature working women. In a regression model, 47% of the variability in retirement attitude is explained by financial planning for retirement, attitude of significant others toward respondent's retirement, attitude toward outside-of-work time, and work commitment.

185   Kaplan, B. (1985). **Women 65 and over: factors associated with their decision to work.** Unpublished doctoral dissertation, Brandeis University, 189p.

Analyzes factors associated with decision of women to work after age 65. Uses data from March 1982 Current Population Survey. Author suggests important policy implications for the labor force participation of older women.

186   Maxwell, S. (1983). **Occupational sex segregation and mobility: analysis of the career experiences of mature women, 1967-1977.** Unpublished doctoral dissertation, Texas A&M University, 222p.

Analyzes the labor experiences of mature women through the empirical examination of their mobility between occupational sectors defined on the basis of sex composition. Based on data from the National Longitudinal Surveys of Work Experience.

187   Oestreich, M. (1984). **Life patterns of middle-aged, working-class women: implications for adult education.** Unpublished doctoral dissertation, The Ohio State University, 134p.

Transitions in the lives of women are related to the circumstances of life rather than to age, such situations as growing independence of children, dissatisfaction with the marriage relationship, desire of women to be financially independent. Women in mid-life look forward to the years ahead of them.

188   Rosen, A. (1982). **Work and general well being of older women.** Unpublished doctoral dissertation, University of Maryland Baltimore Professional Schools, 198p.

Primary purpose of this study was to examine meaning and importance of the work role for older women by looking at differences in general well-being scores between working, nonworking, and retired women aged 45 to 74. The significantly higher general well-being scores of working women over nonworking and retired "reaffirmed the importance of the work role in the lives of older women. Women with higher education and income, white, 60 to 64, and working, were more likely to have high general well-being scores. Women with the lowest education and income levels, black, 45 to 59, retired or nonworking, were likely to have low general well-being scores."

189   Sangster, E. (1984). Older women graduate students: coping patterns in a large university. Unpublished doctoral dissertation, University of Michigan, 178p.

Forty-eight older women graduate students sampled; then 10 case histories developed. Four coping patterns were identified--assertive, manipulative, adaptive, and avoidant.

190   Whitfield, P. (1984). Patterns of success in non-traditionally prepared mature women educational leaders: six case studies. Unpublished doctoral dissertation, Brigham Young University, 273p.

Proposes to offer role models for women, especially those over 40, aspiring to leadership roles in education; to identify who is "there," how they achieved their positions, and how they used this period of their lives as one of generativity rather than one of decline.

Retirement

Books

191   Friedman, R., & Nussbaum, A.   (1986). <u>Coping with your husband's retirement</u>. New York: Simon & Schuster, Inc., 223p.

Interviews with 75 wives of retirees indicate plans for the future of the marriage are as important as financial planning. Guidelines are offered on doing things together and separately, and on avoiding conflicts with regard to housing, finances, travel, and diet.

Articles/chapters

192   Atchley, R. (1982). **The process of retirement: comparing women and men.** In Szinovacz, M. (Ed.), <u>Women's retirement: policy implications of recent research</u>, pp. 158-168. Beverly Hills: Sage Publications, Inc., 271p.

In this study, women not planning to retire generally were unmarried, in average health, and in low-status occupations. For women, the lower the occupational status, the larger the number of expected pensions, and the less positive the attitude toward retirement, the higher the planned age at retirement. Economic aspects of retirement seem to be paramount in deciding to retire later. "Women's attitudes in retirement respond more than men's to ups and downs in circumstances."

193   Coyle, J. (1986). **Retirement planning and the woman business owner.** In Bell, M. J. (Ed.), <u>Women as elders: images, visions, and issues</u>, pp. 51-58. New York: Harrington press, 90p.

Questions on retirement issues relevant to the self-employed woman business owner are discussed.

194   Coyle, J. (1984). Women's attitudes toward planning for retirement. In Bastida, E. (Ed.), Older women: current issues and problems, p. 113-124 of Convergence in Aging, Kansas City, Kansas: Mid-America Congress on Aging, 136p.

The article examines attitudes toward planning for retirement among American women. Secondary analysis of data from the 1974 study by the National Council on the Aging. Finds as the worker role assumes greater importance for women, more information is needed about women's attitudes toward work and toward retirement planning and refining of measures of women's attitudes toward retirement planning.

195   Dorfman, L., & Moffett, M. (1987). Retirement satisfaction in married and widowed rural women. The Gerontologist, 27(2), 215-221.

Married and widowed rural women are compared on retirement satisfaction. For married subjects, financial adequacy, financial frequency, and certainty of aid from friends predict satisfaction. For widowed women, maintenance of preretirement friendships and frequency of visits with friends predict satisfaction.

196   Ekerdt, D. (1987). Retirement. In Maddox, G. (Ed.), The encyclopedia of aging, pp. 577-580. New York: Springer Publishing Company, 890p.

Provides data on U.S. labor force participation rates by gender and age.

197   George, L., Fillenbaum, G., & Palmore, E. (1984). Sex differences in the antecedents and consequences of retirement. The Journal of Gerontology, 39(3), 363-371.

Males and females are compared on antecedents and consequences of retirement. For both groups, retirement had positive and negative effects. Variables predicting retirement for men do not predict retirement for women, and retirement affects substantially more outcomes for men than for women.

198   Gigy, L. (1985-86). Preretired and retired women's attitudes toward retirement. International Journal of Aging and Human Development, 11(1), 31-44.

The focus of this study is on the meaning of retirement for women and on factors associated with adjustment among employed and retired women. The factors associated with psychological functioning may be different before and after retirement.

199   Jewson, R. (1982). After retirement: an exploratory study of the professional woman. In Szinovacz, M. (Ed.), Women's retirement: policy implications of recent research, pp. 169-181. Beverly Hills: Sage Publications, Inc., 271p.

The retiree's perception of herself determines the attitudes of others. "A woman's retirement options may differ from a man's because of societal, institutional, social-psychological, and personality variables. The female may have had more anticipatory socialization for retirement than the male because she has had a homemaker role which continues in retirement   Most female retirees in this study find life more pleasurable in retirement, still feel useful, have a high feeling of purpose, and are quite satisfied with retirement."

200   Kaye, L., & Monk, A. (1984). Sex role traditions and retirement from academe. The Gerontologist, 24(4), 420-426.

The study considers the influence of gender on pre- and post-retirement behavior in academe. Female retirees spend more time in social or recreational activities, make greater use of employer assistance in retirement preparation, and believe more strongly that the university should provide economic and social assistance to employees than do males. Both males and females enjoy their status in retirement.

201   Keith, P. (1985). Work, retirement, and well-being among unmarried men and women. The Gerontologist, 25(4), 410-416.

Evaluations of work, retirement, and well-being of 1,398 never-married, widowed, and divorced/separated males and females find factors associated with evaluations are similar across the three marital statuses. Formerly married women are seen as the most needing of attention from persons planning pre-retirement programs.

202   Newman, E., Sherman, S., & Higgins, C.   (1982).   Retirement expectations and plans: a comparison of professional men and women. In Szinovacz, M. (Ed.), Women's retirement: policy implications of recent research, pp. 113-122. Beverly Hills: Sage Publications, Inc., 271p.

There are small gender differences among professional university or college staff with regard to expectations and plans for retirement.   The implication is that university professionals, especially faculty, want to continue working after their formal retirement, and that "financial issues constitute a major retirement concern even for persons employed in relatively high-level and well-paid occupations."   Retirement preparation programs for younger workers are an option.

203   Prentis, R.   (1980).   White-collar working women's perception of retirement. The Gerontologist, 20(1), 90-95.

A study of 1,235 white-collar working women's views toward retirement finds inadequate preparation for retirement among the subjects. Most subjects look forward to retirement and are confident of making a satisfactory adjustment in retirement.

204   Price-Bonham, S., & Johnson, C. (1982). Attitudes toward retirement: a comparison of professional and nonprofessional married women. In Szinovacz, M. (Ed.), Women's retirement: policy implications of recent research, pp. 123-138. Beverly Hills: Sage Publications, Inc., 271p.

Professional women are less likely to express positive retirement attitudes if they have a lengthy employment history and spend a considerable amount of time with work activities. Professional women who are strongly committed to their work report especially negative retirement attitudes.

205   Seecombe, K., & Lee, G.   (1986).   Gender differences in retirement
        satisfaction and its antecedents. Research on Aging, 8(3), 426-440.

The study examines differences between men and women in levels of self-reported
satisfaction with retirement and in selected antecedents of retirement satisfaction including
health, marital status, occupational status, and income. "Retirement is not a categorically
different experience for women than for men, particularly as retirement satisfaction seems
responsive to the same causes regardless of gender.   The lower levels of retirement
satisfaction among women appear to be due to their lower incomes in retirement and, to a
lesser extent, their lower probabilities of being married."

206   Shaw, L.   (1984).   Retirement plans of middle-aged married women.
        The Gerontologist, 24(2), 154-159.

Husbands' plans have a strong impact on wives' plans for retirement, as does women's own
pension eligibility.

207   Szinovacz, M.   (1983).   Beyond the hearth: older women and
        retirement.   In Markson, E. (Ed.), Older women, pp. 93-120.
        Lexington, Massachusetts: Lexington Books/D.C. Heath & Co., 351p.

Existing studies on female retirement are based on unrepresentative and/or small samples.
Some results are contradictory. Szinovacz says, "These investigations demonstrate beyond
doubt that retirement constitutes an important life event for women that deserves careful
study, that women's retirement needs differ from those of men, that preretirement programs
and   agencies   dealing   with   retirees   will   have   to   take   these   differences   into
consideration...The development of adequate retirement programs for women depends upon
our understanding of this increasingly widespread social phenomenon (i.e., women's
retirement); to acquire such understanding we need additional longitudinal and large-scale
research on women's retirement."

Films

208   Firestone, C. (Producer). (1978). Mountain people. ALMI.

The retirement picture for the elderly of rural Dingess, West Virginia, is shown. A couple
in their eighties and in their seventies exhibit self-sufficiency--they grow food, tend farms,
maintain crafts, hold jobs, and maintain family relationships.

209   Kradlak, C. (Producer). (1978, produced; 1979, released).   A week
        full of Saturdays. Alternate.

The usefulness of preretirement planning is exhibited via several men and women from
different backgrounds discussing housing, finances, family relations, and leisure time
activities.

Dissertations

210   Cassidy, M. (1982). The effects of retirement on emotional well-being:
       a comparison of men and women. Unpublished doctoral dissertation,
       Washington State University, 171p.

Emotional well-being has two elements: self-worth and morale. Retirement negatively
affects the self-worth of women, but not of men, and positively affects the morale of both
men and women. Retirees are more socially active than employed persons, and social
activity enhances emotional well-being.1 Health has the strongest positive direct effect on
emotional well-being, and age has the strongest negative indirect effect on emotional well-
being.

211   Frye, L. (1984). Adjustment to retirement of male and female
       professors. Unpublished doctoral dissertation, The University of
       Wisconsin-Madison, 128p.

The survey of 222 retired professors from the University of Wisconsin-Madison investigates
retirement adjustment.   The personal interviews included a 20% female sample.
Relationships are found between morale and both variables of adjustment to retirement.
Preretirement feeling is statistically significant on one dependent variable and preretirement
feeling, reason for retirement, financial planning for retirement, and health are statistically
significantly affected by the other dependent variable.

212   Liss, B. (1982). Life satisfaction: a comparison of retired and
       employed women. Unpublished doctoral dissertation, University of
       Texas Health Science Center at Houston, 172p.

The focus is on life satisfaction for retired and employed women with long-term
employment in a typically female occupational setting. The retired subjects' perceptions of
their health and social participation are more positive than the employed women's.
Traditional retired women demonstrated higher life satisfaction than nontraditional retired
women. Both retired and employed women who perceive continuity in life patterns score
statistically higher on life satisfaction than women who perceive discontinuity. Financial
planning is the area of greatest retirement concern for retired and employed women.

213   Madigan, M. (1985). Preparation for prime time: three business
       women at work and in retirement. Unpublished doctoral dissertation,
       Columbia University Teachers College, 194p.

An ethnographic study of the first retirement year of three business women of varied
employment and marital status shows the impact on choices of the three on satisfaction
with retirement decision and lifestyle.   "They believed the combination of economic
security and personal support systems eased the transition from work to retirement."

214   Rotman, A. (1981). Professional women in retirement. Unpublished
       doctoral dissertation, University of Pittsburgh, 271p.

This study of the impact of midlife family responsibilities on retirement adjustment and
flexibility (experience in coping with change) of professional women examines involvement
with family, work, and leisure in two timeframes--during the peak period of family

responsibilities and in retirement. Among the findings are that women with a high degree of family responsibilities have negative attitudes toward retirement and positive feelings of morale. There is no correlation between the two scales measuring retirement attitudes and morale.

Health

Books

215   Ammer, C.   (1983).   The A to Z of women's health.   New York: Everest House, 481p.

This textbook of obstetrics and gynecology is written in understandable English, with "insights, lore, and treatments of the feminist clinics and a smattering of general medicine." Written with underlying assumption "that every woman wants to take responsibility for her own health, and the only way she can act intelligently and safely in her own best interest is to understand the working of her body and to know what kinds of care and treatment are available." Attempt has been made to present all sides of controversial questions.

216   Anderson, L.   (1984).   Aging and loneliness: an international study of a group of elderly women.   Stockholm: Department of Psychosocial Environmental Medicine, Karolinska Institute, 174p.

Among 207 elderly women living in Stockholm, Sweden, aged 16 to 74, differences in loneliness were not great.

217   Birren, J., & Moore, J.   (1975).   The relation of stress and age.   Los Angeles: Ethel Percy Andrus Gerontology Center, University of Southern California, 50p.

Sections on widowhood, male and female differences, and midlife crisis.

218   Budoff, P.   (1983).   No more hot flashes, and other good news.   New York: Putnam, 272p.

Focus on getting preventive medical care, what to do for medical problems, and how to get help. Includes chapters on hormone-replacement therapy, ovarian cancer, urinary tract infection, and laboratory tests.

219   Doress, P. et al. (1987). Ourselves, growing older: women aging with knowledge and power. New York: Simon & Schuster, 511p.

Discusses health and living issues of midlife and older women.   Reports personal experiences of women and the views of experts on such topics as aging and well-being, body image, sexuality, relationships, work and retirement, living arrangements, money matters, and medical problems.

220   Edelstein, B. (1982). The woman doctor's medical guide for women. New York: Morrow, 310p.

Explains what changes to expect in one's body (with aging) and how to cope with them; diseases and how to keep risks; when drugs can help; dealing with psychological traumas; and coping with obesity.

221   Egginton, M., Kunigonis, M., Mintz, J., & Roser, D. (1984). An older woman's health guide. New York: McGraw-Hill Book co., 260p.

Practical information on social and family relationships, alternative approaches to health care, mental health goals, maintaining wellness.

222   Franks, V., & Rothblum, E. (Eds.). (1983). The stereotyping of women: its effects on mental health. New York: Springer Publishing Co., 275p.

Describes the prevalence of disorders such as depression and agoraphobia, especially emphasizing women and these disorders, relates sex-role stereotypes to the   disorders, delineates research on women in each area of mental health, and describes "future implications for research and intervention in women's mental health."   Sections detail relationship of sex-role stereotypes and health, conceptual models of sex-role stereotypes, language use, stereotyping by children, depression, agoraphobia, assertiveness, sexual dysfunction, weight, and violence.

223   Golub, S., & Freedman, R. (Eds.). (1985). Health needs of women as they age. New York: Haworth Press, 122p.

Focus by 10 contributors on the health care needs of women as they mature beyond middle age--common health problems for women as they age, how their needs are being met, and what problems are not being adequately addressed by the medical care system.

224   Haug, M., Ford, A., & Sheafor, M. (Eds.). (1985). The physical and mental health of aged women. New York: Springer Publishing Company, 303p.

Integrates behavioral and medical perspectives of the mental, physical and living problems, strengths, and coping abilities of older women. Women's common physical and biological makeup may be one factor in their longevity, currently an average life expectancy exceeding that of males by about five years.

225   Henig, R. (1985). How a woman ages. New York: Esquire Press, 272p.

Presents scientific and medical evidence for a hopeful view of aging, describes predictable changes after 30 and what can be done to stave off or ameliorate age-related disorders, recognizing the symptoms of aging for what they are.

226   Lake, A. (1979). Our own years: what women over 35 should know about themselves. New York: CBS Publications, 243p.

A pragmatic approach to changes occurring with normal aging for women. Focuses on menopause, sexual relations, physical fitness, health, the heart, cancer, weight, changes in skin, hair, the back, bones, eyes, teeth, and memory, stress. Concludes with facts and futuristic predictions. One crucial research finding reported is that the experience of men and women, through life's stages, is profoundly different. "Midlife is the stage when men may suffer crisis and women experience fruition."

227   Millette, B., & Hawkins, J. (1983). Women and the menopause: a book for and about women and the climacteric. Reston, Virginia: Reston Publishing Col., 148p.

A time of transition, menopause is seen as a developmental life event. Discusses health care, myths and fantasies about sex and the menopause.

228   Nudel, A. (1978). For the woman over 50: a practical guide for a full and vital life. New York: Taplinger Publishing Co., Inc., 436p.

Manual of facts on topics ranging from the estrogen replacement controversy to proposed national health insurance to body image to emotional accessibility to career strategies to retirement preparation.   Written for the woman over 50 with direct, specific factual information about major areas of life concern, with sensible options and suggestions.

Articles/chapters

229   Berkun, C. (1983). Changing appearance for women in the middle years of life: trauma. In Markson, E. (Ed.), Older women, pp. 11-35. Lexington, Massachusetts: Lexington Books/D. C. Heath & Co., 351p.

Author concludes that middle-aged women's behavior patterns and values, likely to fit the feminine stereotype, may be dysfunctional for them in middle age.

230   Berry, J., Storandt, M., & Coyne, A. (1984). Age and sex differences in somatic complaints associated with depression. The Journal of Gerontology, 29(4), 465-467.

Reports that somatic complaints are especially prominent in older women. Older women, compared with younger women, reported greater difficulty sleeping at night, less interest in sex, loss of appetite, and increased constipation. The authors suggest that these somatic complaints are similar to physical changes accompanying the aging process and these problems should be explored before attributing them to a depressive disorder.

231   Campbell, S. (1983-84). The 50-year-old woman and midlife stress. International Journal of Aging and Human Development, 18(4), 295-307.

Women in their fifties are susceptible to many internal and external stresses--e.g., widowhood, divorce, poverty. The author suggests obstacles to successful aging and coping techniques.

232   Cohen, D., Schaie, K., & Gribbin, K. (1977). The organization of spatial abilities in older men and women. The Journal of Gerontology, 32(5), 578-585.

"Men and women appear to have the same cognitive structure with no differences between the sexes on the latent constructs." Tests of spatial ability seem "to underestimate performance on the latent construct of spatial ability in women and on the latent construct of verbal ability in men."

233   DeLorey, C. (1984). Health care and midlife women. In Baruch, G., & Brooks-Gunn, J. (Eds.), Women in midlife, pp. 277-301. New York: Plenum Press, 404p.

Discussion of health care for midlife women, taking into account how the health care system functions and the need to understand the totality of women's health experiences.

234   Engle, V., & Graney, M. (1985-86). Self-assessed and functional health of older women. International Journal of Aging and Human Development, 22(4), 301-313.

Significant correlations to self-assessment of health were found among measures of functional health, self-concept and attitudes, and demographic variables, such as body care and movement, emotional behavior activities, age self-concept, self-assessment of speed, and identity as a homemaker.

235   Kannel, W., & Brand, F. (1983). Cardiovascular risk factors in the elderly. In Markson, E. (Ed.), Older women, pp. 315-327. Lexington, Massachusetts: Lexington Books/D. C. Heath & Co., 351p.

Much of this chapter was based on findings in the Framingham Epidemiological Heart Disease Study. Among women, "distinct tendency for the proportionate mortality attributed to cardiovascular disease to increase with age...coronary heart disease increases with age for women accounts for the highest incidence of cardiovascular events among them."

236   Kerzner, L. (1983). Physical changes after menopause. In Markson, E. (Ed.), Older women, pp. 299-313. Lexington, Massachusetts: Lexington Books/D. C. Heath & Co., 351p.

Discusses the physical changes which affect women as they age, such as menopause, cardiovascular disease, falls and fractures, osteoporosis, and estrogen use.

237   Krause, N. (1986). Stress and sex differences in depressive symptoms among older adults. The Journal of Gerontology, 41(6), 727-731.

Investigates whether elderly men or women experience more symptoms associated with depression, and, if sex differences exist, what factors might account for the greater preponderance of psychological distress among women. Random community survey of 351 older adults. Greater vulnerability among women to the effects of chronic life strains explained a substantial portion of the observed sex differences in distress.

238   Levy, S. (1980-81). The adjustment of the older woman: effects of chronic ill health and attitudes toward retirement. International Journal of Aging and Human Development, 12(2), 93-110.

Healthy and ill females who had not wanted to retire did not adjust, over time, to retirement.

239   Lohr, M., Essex, M., & Klein, M. (1988). The relationships of coping responses to physical health status and life satisfaction among older women. The Journal of Gerontology, 43(2), P54-P60.

Examines a model of the causal links among physical, functional, and subjective aspects of physical health and life satisfaction among older women. Investigates the effects of three coping responses--direct-action, positive-cognitive, and passive-cognitive.

240   Markson, E. (1985-86). Gender roles and memory loss in old age: an exploration of linkages. International Journal of Aging and Human Development, 22(3), 205-214.

Case study of relationship between self-preoccupation, group affiliation, object relations, and memory loss among three older working-class women. Found that a high frequency of self-references in speech indicated memory loss and less attention to present experience.

241   Melick, M., & Logue, J. (1985-86). The effect of disaster on the health and well-being of older women. International Journal of Aging and Human Development, 21(1), 27-38.

A retrospective cohort survey was carried out five years after a major flood in the Wyoming Valley of Pennsylvania, with a subsample of women 65 and over used in this analysis. Significant differences occurred in self-perceptions, including state of mind after the flood, distress during recovery, quality of life after the flood, and frequency of thinking about the flood activities.

242   McIntosh, J., & Santos, J. (1985-86). Methods of suicide by age: sex
      and race differences among the young and old. International Journal
      of Aging and Human Development, 212(2), 123-139.

The elderly have the highest suicide rate in the United States. This study investigated age-
sex-race groups, trends over time, and methods of suicide used. Women use the more
lethal methods less often than men and less lethal methods more often than men, but the
differences are not as great as they once were.

243   Ory, M., & Goldberg, E. (1983). Pet possession and well-being in
      elderly women. Research on Aging, 5(3), 389-409.

Pet ownership seen as an independent predictor of perceived happiness in elderly women.
Preliminary finding is that a large percentage of women who are not very attached to their
pets are unhappy, compared to women who are very attached to their pets or even those
with no pets at all.

244   Ridley, J., Bachrach, C., & Dawson, D. (1979). Recall and reliability
      of interview data from older women. The Journal of Gerontology,
      34(1), 99-105.

Retrospective fertility histories from women in birth cohorts of 1901-1910 (aged 66 to 76)
were used. Subjects answered exactly on an average of 90 percent of questions they were
asked.

245   Rikli, R., & Busch, S. (1986). Motor performance of women as a
      function of age and physical activity level. The Journal of Gerontology,
      41(5), 645-649.

Older active women were compared with older inactive men, and active and inactive
younger women on reaction time, balance, and flexibility. Except for grip strength, scores
of older active women on all measures were significantly better than for older inactive
women, and much more like those of the younger women.

246   Sinnott, J. (1984-85). Stress, health, and mental health symptoms of
      older women and men. International Journal of Aging and Human
      Development, 20(2), 123-132.

Examined mental health scores, stress, and health. Average woman tested described more
symptoms [than did the average man]. Her symptoms were related to health (including
doctor visits), but not to age or stress and conflict.

247   Verbrugge, L. (1984). A health profile of older women with
      comparisons to older men. Research on Aging, 6(3), 291-322.

Compares physical health status of women 65 and over to older men using data from
ongoing national health surveys and vital statistics. Older women were found to be more
frequently ill than older men, with both acute and chronic conditions, but their problems
were found to be less life-threatening than men's.

248   Verbrugge, L. (1987). Sex differences in health. In Maddox, G. (Ed.),
       The encyclopedia of aging, pp. 601-604. New York: Springer
       Publishing Company, 890p.

Women have a longevity advantage over men. Older males and females have similar
evaluations of their health status. Older women have higher rates for many more chronic
conditions, but older men have more serious chronic problems.

Films

249   Bloom, A. (Producer). (1975). Virginia. DIRECT.

Presents a portrait of Virginia, an elderly woman with a hearing handicap. Shows her
patience, gentleness, and triumph over her handicap.

250   Brown, S. (Producer). (No date). Menopause: a time of transition.
       Planned Parenthood of Alameda/San Francisco.

Provides information to eliminate the fears and worry often accompanying menopause.

251   Burnford, Z., & Burnford, P. (Producers). (1980). Menopause:
       myths and realities. (Also video).

Attitude is seen to be a key to accepting the changes normally occurring during menopause.
Six women who are experiencing menopause describe how they are dealing with this
normal process of life.

252   Carnochan, D. (Producer). Memaw.

Filmed on last day which Memaw, 88, who has Alzheimer's, spends on her farm. "The
day marks a passage in the lives of Memaw, her daughter, and granddaughter as well as
the 200-year-old farm" and portrays the dilemma faced by many people with aging parents.

253   Chase, D. (1983). Glass curtain.

Dramatization of a woman's struggles to cope with the Alzheimer's disease of her mother.

254   Feil, E. (1981). One hundred years to live.

A woman and her mother evidence mental and physical deterioration after moving to a
nursing home.

255   Kungle, M., & Welshufer, J.   (1983).   Planning to maintain independence: Mrs. Armstrong's case.   Video Resources Library, University of Wisconsin-Madison.

Steps involved in home care for an older woman.

256   Maryland, University of.   (1984).   Dominick and Margaret: independence--a way of life.

Illustrates how Margaret McCullough and Dominick Ciamarra, two elderly, handicapped persons live independently after they have overcome social, physical, and psychological problems.

257   McCallum, E. (1983). Brittle bones. Filmakers Library.

Explains osteoporosis, which affects 25% of women over the age of 60.   Personal experiences of victims and discussion of new discoveries and treatment.

258   Menopause. (1983).

Presents a detailed explanation of the menopausal experience of an individual woman. Realistic seminar discussion of eight other women discussing their menopause.

259   Oliva, M. (Producer). (1982). Beware: the gaps in medical care for older people.

Depicts a family's concern for Beatrice, 78, a depressed woman, who has been hospitalized after a fall and again after a severe emotional episode.   The films discusses over-medication, stereotypes, and the need for special knowledge in treating older people.

260   Robertson, T. (Producer). (1982). Grandma didn't wave back. (Video).

Illustrates 11-year-old Debbie's confusion as her grandmother's senility worsens.

261   Rubbo, M., & Walker, G. (1983). Daisy: the story of a facelift. National Film Board of Canada.

Follows a woman having a facelift from planning through the recovery period.

262   Video Services. (1983). Living with Grace.

Shows everyday life of an Alzheimer's victim.

263   Washington, University of, Press. (1982). **Aging and health in a five generation American family.** (Video).

Various parts of human life span are represented by women aged 87, 69, 51, 27, 4.

Documents

264   Davis, L., & Brody, E. (1979). **Rape and older women.** Rockville, Maryland: U.S. Department of Health, Education, and Welfare, Public Health Service, Alcohol, Drug Abuse, and Mental Health Administration, National Institute of Mental Health, 171p.

Discussion of the special vulnerability of older women and the physical and psychological impact which fear of crime and sexual assault have on the lifestyle of older women. Suggested avoidance activities. Outline of educational and training tools for older women, community groups, etc.

265   Endicott, J. (1986). **Premenstrual changes, syndromes, and disorders.** Women's Mental Health Occasional Paper Series, National Institute of Mental Health, United States Department of Health and Human Services, 21p.

A call for investigators and clinicians to address the diversity of patterns in premenstrual changes, syndromes, and disorders rather than global measures of "a premenstrual syndrome," consciousness of patient's ongoing mental or medical disorders, and awareness (by patients) of cyclical mood and behavior changes.

266   Gelfand, D. (1983). **Working paper No. 5--mental health concerns of older women.** University of Maryland, College Park, Maryland, National Policy Center on Women and Aging, 58p.

Questions extent to which diagnoses reflect biases of mental health professionals. Covers mental health classifications, prevalence of disorders among older women and mental health policy; presents alternatives which can ameliorate the mental health concerns of older women.

267   Health and Human Services, U.S. Department of. (1987). **Health resources for older women.** Washington, D.C.: National Institutes of Health, 76p.

This book is "intended as a resource tool for women seeking information or locating services for better medical and health care." Topics covered include age changes and health promotion, common disorders of later life (such as osteoporosis and urinary incontinence), and taking charge (in such areas as housing options, financial planning, and widowhood).

268   Hing, E. (1981). Use of health services by women 65 years and over.
        Hyattsville, Maryland: United States Department of Health and
        Human Services, Public Health Service, Office of Health Research,
        Statistics, and Technology, National Center for Health Statistics, 72p.

Data from the National Health Survey, Series 13, No. 59, are presented. "Major health
characteristic of older women is the greater prevalence of chronic illnesses that cause
limitations in how they live, and these are often multiple in number. The health problems
of aging women are similar to those of aging men, but older women live longer, which
means that they endure these chronic conditions longer."

269   Stone, R. (1984). The effects of retirement on the health status of
        older unmarried women. University of California San Francisco, Aging
        Health Policy Center, 89p.

Explores effects of retirement on the self-assessed health, functional health, and life
satisfaction of a cohort of older unmarried women. In general, there was a gradual decline
in self-assessed health and functional health over the ten-year period, but level of life
satisfaction seemed to stabilize after 1975.

270   U.S. Congress. House. Subcommittee on Health and Long-term care
        and the Task Force on Social Security and Women of the Select
        Committee on Aging. 99th Congress. (1986). Breast cancer detection:
        the need for a federal response. 169p.

Prevention and health maintenance seen as crucial for women after 65, as they are earlier in
women's lives.

271   U.S. Congress. House. Task Force on Social Security and Women of
        Subcommittee on Retirement Income and Employment and Select
        Committee on Aging. 99th Congress. (1986). Older women's health.
        67p.

Health care of older women--accessibility and developing trends--seen as a primary concern
for 18 million elderly women in the United States.

272   U.S. Congress. Senate. Special Committee on Aging. 99th Congress.
        (1985). Prospects for better health for older women. 71p.

Health care seen as especially important to women because they live longer than men,
suffer more illnesses, have more days of disability, and have more chance of developing
multiple illnesses. Discussion of access to healthy care, health prevention, health education,
caregiving, and technological advances.

Dissertations

273   Alldredge-Marshall, G. (1984). Life satisfaction in aging Americans:
      a causal model. Unpublished doctoral dissertation, Brigham Young
      University, number of pages not given.

Path analysis on relationship of life satisfaction to five other variables--data from National
Opinion Research Center.   For females, health, formal activity, and education had
significant direct effects on life satisfaction.

274   Belgrave, L. (1985). The experience of chronic disease in the everyday
      lives of elderly women. Unpublished doctoral dissertation, Case
      Western Reserve University, 226p.

This study focuses on elderly women with arthritis or diabetes, approaching chronic disease
as an inherently physical problem with social consequences.   Ways of living with chronic
disease included accepting it as a problem to be dealt with, lowering expectations, concern
with physical problems dominating everyday life.

275   Brown, R. (1985). Effects of a strength training program on strength,
      body composition, and self-concept of females. Unpublished doctoral
      dissertation, Brigham Young University, 92p.

Both mature and young females in experimental groups showed increased strength and
improved self-concept, compared to control groups.   Results "support the inclusion of
strength training in fitness programs for healthy mature women and suggest the
effectiveness of strength training in improving the psychological well-being of women."

276   Carr, M. (1985). The effects of aging and depression on time
      perspective in women. Unpublished doctoral dissertation, Columbia
      University, 133p.

Eighty women, aged 50 to 63 and 65 to 89 were included in the study.   There were no
significant differences among the groups on time span, temporal orientation, or perceived
consistency of self-concept. Significant differences in self-esteem were found only between
members of the depressed and nondepressed groups.

277   Cokin, L. (1982). Educated women in their thirties: an exploratory
      psychosocial study. Unpublished doctoral dissertation, The George
      Washington University, 183p.

Explores formation of the early adult life structure in women during the decade between 30
and 450.   Thirties were found to be years for exploration, growth, and change, and for
individuation within the context of relationships to others.

278   Craven, R. (1984). <u>Preventing falls: an educational intervention to increase confidence and safety among elderly women.</u> Unpublished doctoral dissertation, Seattle University, 136p.

Investigated whether elderly women perceived a change in their feelings of confidence and safety after an educational intervention that taught changes in motor stability, environmental and personal hazards, and methods for compensating to prevent falls. Data showed trends toward increases in perceptions of safety and confidence.

279   Eggers, J. (1986). <u>Well-elderly women's entrance and adherence to structured physical fitness programs.</u> Unpublished doctoral dissertation, University of Cincinnati, 120p.

Identified needs and attitudes of well-elderly women about their fitness and about fitness programs to determine how to promote use by well-elderly women of structured physical fitness programs.

280   Fitting, M. (1984). <u>Caregivers for dementia patients: a comparison of men and women.</u> Unpublished doctoral dissertation, University of Denver, 182p.

Comparison of sex and age differences among caregivers for dementia patients. Male and female caregivers similar as caregivers.

281   Friedman, S. (1982). <u>The effect of physical impairment on the social participation patterns of the urban aged.</u> Unpublished doctoral dissertation, University of California, Riverside, 203p.

Examines relationship between physical impairment and social participation among urban aged persons. Sex, age, religion, ethnicity, and distance from children were variables included in the models.

282   Goldberg, S. (1985). <u>An investigation into the usefulness of gender typing as a construct in understanding self-esteem in old age.</u> Unpublished doctoral dissertation, Temple University, 177p.

Androgynous individuals were found to have the highest level of self-esteem among these subjects.

283   Hupp, S. (1985). <u>Satisfaction of older women in leisure programs: an investigation of contributing factors.</u> Unpublished doctoral dissertation, University of Oregon, 136p.

Study of relationship of leisure satisfaction and leisure attitude to leisure program satisfaction of 294 women 55 and older.

284   Johnson, S. (1982). <u>Time-series analysis of individual performances of older women on a serial gross motor task.</u> Unpublished doctoral dissertation, The University of North Carolina, 312p.

Study of memory for movement sequences and relative importance of visual and kinesthetic information for motor performance of four right-handed females, aged 61 to 75.

285   Kennedy, C. (1982). <u>An examination of the relative strength of health as a predictor of life satisfaction of the elderly.</u> Unpublished doctoral dissertation, The University of Toledo, 126p.

Six hundred and thirty-eight females were included in this study, which found that perceived health and life satisfaction were significantly related even when controlling for sex, race, and income.

286   Kopac, C. (1985). <u>A study of the relationships between personal characteristics, life events, the environment, the Type A behavior pattern, and well-being in older persons.</u> Unpublished doctoral dissertation, University of Maryland, 328p.

The Type A behavior pattern was predictive of illness in this aged sample. For men, religious intrinsic motivation, uncontrolled life events, and past occupation were associated with illness in old age, while, for women, a decline in socializing was associated with illness and with a decrease in happiness; increased uncontrolled life events were associated with decreased functional status and a decline in happiness; advancing age was associated with a decline in functional status. Uncontrolled life events were associated with illness and a decline in functional status for both men and women.

287   Langford, J. (1985). <u>Life satisfaction of elderly persons with mental retardation living in care centers.</u> Unpublished doctoral dissertation, University of Utah, 234p.

This study focused on life satisfaction of elderly mentally retarded persons. Demographic data revealed that the average resident with mental retardation is a 67-year-old, white, single woman who lived in an intermediate care facility for the mentally retarded just prior to her current residence and had been institutionalized for over 28 years in a state training school.

288   Lasser, S. (1984). <u>Adjustment to cardiac illness: the effects of age, gender, and socioeconomic status.</u> Unpublished doctoral dissertation, St. John's University, 347p.

Relationship of subjects' compliance to medical regimens, perceptions of care, role change, work resumption, and effects of the social network system to age, sex, and socioeconomic status. Twelve males, twenty females, aged 39 to 65, with myocardial infarction or angina pectoris within the previous six months to two years were the subjects. Based on comparisons of their accounts, they were categorized into "resenters," "strugglers," and "accommodators."

289   Lesser, M. (1984). <u>Anxiety levels of younger and older women in their first term pregnancies.</u> Unpublished doctoral dissertation, University of Miami, 135p.

Comparison of differences in anxiety levels of first pregnancies of women 19-24, 25-29, 30 and older. There were no significant differences in trait anxiety as a function of age.

290   Louie, D. (1984). Sex difference in the life experience-depression relationship among the elderly. Unpublished doctoral dissertation, Syracuse University, 234p.

National random sample of 521 community elderly 65 and older in 1968 and 1971. Life experience is different for men and women, both quantitatively and qualitatively. The mean psychiatric symptomatology, life events, and social support for women is higher than for men.

291   Luggen, A. (1985). The pain experience of ten selected elderly women. Unpublished doctoral dissertation, University of Cincinnati, 268p.

Ten elderly widows, with low incomes, relatively asocial or moderately so, moderately depressed with high intensity of pain during most of their waking hours, used few medications. Their instruments were prayer, hoping, and coping self-statements.

292   Manzella, D. (1982). Activity patterns of hearing impaired elderly women. Unpublished doctoral dissertation, University of California, Los Angeles, 123p.

Explores, through retrospective analysis, sample of 15 healthy elderly women, if elderly women with hearing loss report significant changes in their life patterns because of their hearing loss, and whether these women have made adjustments in their behavior to compensate for their hearing loss. These women did not, and have not, experienced significant changes in the way they relate to others.

293   McGloshen, T. (1985). Factors related to the psychological well-being of elderly recent widows. Unpublished doctoral dissertation, The Ohio State University, 84p.

Of 226 women 60 or older, widowed for 7 to 21 months, those widows who were healthy and active (especially in religious activities), had not worked outside the home during their marriages, had not had earlier experiences with grief, and had husbands who died close to home showed higher psychological well-being than other widows.

294   McLaughlin, W. (1984). The effects of an age-specific exercise program on aerobic capacity, body composition, body-image, and exercise behavior in 42-77-year-old women. Unpublished doctoral dissertation, University of Maryland, 183p.

Aerobic capacity and body composition were not significant predictors of body-image and all three of these variables were not significant predictors of exercise behavior among the middle-aged and older women in this study.

295   Nagy, M. (1982). Attributional differences in health status and life satisfactions of older women: a comparison between widows and non-widows. Unpublished doctoral dissertation, University of Oregon, 150p.

The objective of this research was to determine if widows 55 and over differed from married women in the same age group on their life satisfaction and health status. Both groups were satisfied and happy.

296   Obear, M.   (1985).   The nutritional status of a group of elderly
       institutionalized women: relationships to stress and social support.
       Unpublished doctoral dissertation, State University of New York at
       Buffalo, 254p.

Examined relationships among nutritional status, dietary intake, stress, and social support in
a sample of well elderly women living in a long-term care institution.

297   Saalwaechter, K. (1983).   Effects of three counseling modalities on self-
       concept of older women.   Unpublished doctoral dissertation, Memphis
       State University, 83p.

Study to determine effects of verbal, tactile, and verbal/tactile counseling modalities on
particular aspects of self-concept of single women age 65 and older living independently.

298   Sommers, T. (1982).   Age differences in recall and recognition memory
       of young and elderly adults as a function of type of stimuli and length
       of retention interval.   Unpublished doctoral dissertation, The University
       of Toledo, 108p.

Age, type of stimuli, and retention interval play important roles in recall and recognition
performance, with young subjects doing better than elderly subjects.

299   Weaver, D. (1984).   A study to determine the effect of exercise on
       depression in middle-aged women.   Unpublished doctoral dissertation,
       Middle Tennessee State University, 180p.

Study of effects of aerobic exercise on emotional depression among middle-aged women.
An aerobic exercise program was found to be an effective method of alleviating depression
in middle-aged women.

Sexuality

Books

300 Fuchs, E. (1977). <u>The second season: life, love, and sex--women in the middle years</u>. Garden City, New York: Anchor Press/Doubleday, 298p.

This book is "designed to present a rational, enlightened view of the physiological and cross-cultural components of women's experience with middle age and the universal fact of menopause." The focus is on menopause, sexuality, hysterectomy, divorce and widowhood, pregnancy, and the multiple roles of women. Chapter reference notes and "A Shopper's Guide to Surgery" are included.

301 Wharton, G. (1981). <u>Sexuality and aging: an annotated bibliography</u>. Metuchen, New Jersey, and London: The Scarecrow Press, Inc., 251p.

Major works about the sexual activity of older persons are identified.

Articles

302 Damrosch, S. (1984). Graduate nursing students' attitudes toward sexually active older persons. <u>The Gerontologist</u>, <u>24</u>(3), 299-302.

Graduate nursing students in the sample showed bias favoring a sexually active 68-year-old woman on such variables as adjustment and cheerfulness.

303 Luria, Z., & Meade, R. (1984). Sexuality and the middle-aged woman. In Baruch, G., & Brooks-Gunn, J. (Eds.). <u>Women in Midlife</u>, pp. 371-397. New York: Plenum Press, 404p.

The chapter looks at research evidence on sexuality of women aged 40 to 60. Recent changes in women's sexual behavior indicate that female sexuality does not exist only as an adjunct to romantic love. Little is known about the meanings of specific sexual acts in women's lives. What is known about women's experience of being sexual in midlife depends on the women's age cohort, marital status, and the measure of being sexual used in a given study.

304   Starr, B. (1987). Sexuality. In Maddox, G. (Ed.), The encyclopedia of aging, pp. 606-608. New York: Springer Publishing Company, 890p.

In their mid-thirties, women reach a sexual response peak, which remains at that level throughout the rest of their lives. While a common stereotype is that menopause reduces sexuality, "most older women report feeling sexually liberated after menopause."

305   Stimson, A., Wase, J., & Stimson, J. (1981). Sexuality and self-esteem among the aged. Research on Aging, 3(2), 228-239.

Similar emotional and attitudinal factors underlie integrations of sexuality and self-evaluations for [an earlier study of] college-aged students and [those in this study]. Standards and reference models from youth to old age seem to have different effects on men and women. An active sex life appears to be crucial to an older man's feelings of self-worth and his feelings that he is respected by his friends and secure socially. Dissatisfaction with sexual activity is related to depression and feelings of worthlessness. For older women sexual behavior is a separate activity dimension. "The older woman feels unattractive and therefore socially rejected and of less value," while a younger woman feels confident because she feels attractive.

306   Turner, B., & Adams, C. (1983). The sexuality of older women. In Markson, E. (Ed.), Older women, pp. 55-72. Lexington, Massachusetts: Lexington Books/D. C. Heath & Co., 351p.

The focus is on how the sexuality of women is influenced by gender (the social-psychological dimension of sex status) and by aging. To set in context, "it appears that patterns of sexual behavior and attitudes about sexuality are more variable among women than among men at all ages." Positive change in sexuality is possible, whatever an individual's age. Experience may be more important than changes brought about by physiological aging.

Films

307   Productions Bella (Producer). (1976). One more winter.

Francoise Sagan's vignette of an older couple's romance is presented.

Documents

308   National Institute on Aging, National Institutes of Health, Public Health Service, United States Department of Health and Human Services. (1981). Age page: sexuality in later life, 1p.

Women generally experience little serious loss of sexual capability because of age alone. "Public acceptance of sexuality in later life is gradually increasing."

Dissertations

309 Florence, M. (1983). A survey of sexual learning interests in an older adult population. Unpublished doctoral dissertation, University of Pennsylvania, 320p.

Older adults may be interested in sexual functioning as a part of their total health maintenance. Sexual attitudes do not remain stable through life, but may adjust to environmental factors, such as pressure from their children to accept an expanded view of acceptable sexual behavior and cultural norms.

310 Meske, R. (1983). Personal and sociological factors influencing sexual activity in late-life women. Unpublished doctoral dissertation, The Fielding Institute, 143p.

The author examines certain personal and sociological factors influencing heterosexual desire and activity in 73 women, aged 60 to 89 years. Two factors positively related to higher level of desire and activity with regard to sexual intercourse are living with the opposite sex (in each case married and living with her spouse) and perception of father's attitude toward sex to have been positive. The conclusion of this study is that "decline in, or maintenance of, sexual desire and activity in the late-life woman may have more to do with personal and sociological factors than biological aging."

311 Weinstein, E. (1983). The sexual attitudes, interests and activities of senior adults residing in age-integrated and age-segregated communities. Unpublished doctoral dissertation, Hofstra University, 152p.

This study examines whether middle income older adults residing in age-segregated, leisure-type retirement communities exhibit greater sexual interest and sexual activity and more liberal sexual attitudes than do middle income adults residing in age- integrated mainstream communities.

Religion

Books

312   Cook, S. (1982). <u>I'm no spring chicken, but it's fun being over 40.</u>
Eugene, Oregon: Harvest House Publishers, 128p.

A humorous, religious perspective on women over 40 is presented.

313   Murphy, S. (1983). <u>Midlife wanderer: the woman religious in midlife
transition.</u> Whitinsville, Massachusetts: Affirmation Books, 1983, 175p.

This study of over 200 nuns in midlife represents a three-year investigation of the
experiences of women religious of the midlife transition.   On adult developmental life
tasks, women religious are more androgynous than women or men in general, and similar
to women in general in approximate onset of the midlife transition, emotional experiences
of the transition, intimacy/sexuality concerns, and identity issues. They are similar to men
in general vocational development, career adjustment, and mentoring experiences.

Articles

314   Ainlay, S., & Smith, D.   (1984).   Aging and religious participation.
<u>The Journal of Gerontology,</u> <u>39</u>(3), 357-363.

This article explores religious practices and the aging process.   There is increasing
homogeneity of attitudes and behaviors with increasing age.

315   Alston, L., & Alston, J. (1980). Religion and the older woman. In
Fuller, M., & Martin, C.   (Eds.), <u>The older woman,</u> pp. 262-278.
Springfield, Illinois: Charles C Thomas, Publisher, 343p.

This chapter focuses on whether or not life-cycle stages influence religious behavior.
Today's older woman is likely to be a frequent church attender more so than the older man

or the younger woman. "Women are more religiously active than men at all ages and the more frequent attendance of women is highly correlated with their greater identification with their religious affiliation."

316   Blazer, D., & Palmore, E. (1980). Religion and aging in a longitudinal
       panel. In Fuller, M., & Martin, C. (Eds.), The older woman, pp. 279-
       285. Springfield, Illinois: Charles C Thomas, Publisher, 343p.

Data represent part of the first longitudinal study of aging at Duke University. Women were found to be significantly more religious than men in activities and in attitudes. Religious activity among females remained significantly higher than that for males over time, but declined gradually but definitely over time [as it did for males]. Women and individuals in nonmanual occupations tended to be more religious both in activity and in attitudes.

317   Hunsberger, B. (1985). Religion, age, life satisfaction, and perceived
       sources of religiousness. The Journal of Gerontology, 40(4), 615-620.

This research supports previous findings of a tendency toward increased religiosity in older age. Highly religious older persons report an increase in religiousness over the course of their lives, while subjects low in religiosity tend to report a decrease. Mothers had the strongest proreligious influence on these subjects.

318   Kivett, V. (1979). Religious motivation in middle age: correlates and
       implications. The Journal of Gerontology, 34(1), 106-115.

Three hundred males and females, 45 to 65, from United Methodist churches, comprise the sample for this study. "Women, persons who have high idealized self-concepts, and adults who believe that what happens to them is under their personal control are less likely than others to be extrinsically motivated or to show a self-centered dependence upon religion...An important relationship may exist between the comfort or challenge functions of religion and spiritual well-being in later life for middle-aged groups."

319   Margraff, R. (1986). Aging: religious sisters facing the future. In
       Bell, M. J. (Ed.), Women as elders: images, visions, and issues, pp. 35-
       49. New York: Harrington Press, 90p.

Three congregations of religious women are considered in terms of retirement and value of work, career changes, housing, medical issues, and economic concerns. Decreased entry of young women into religious orders and life expectancy of women in religious orders being above that of the general population--both are leading to disproportionately large aged populations among many orders. The author indicates that there is needed a process to assist individual sisters in planning and taking responsibility for their own old age and that ways should be found for a limited number of sisters to support larger numbers of older sisters whose financial resources are minimal.

320   Taylor, R., & Chatters, L. (1986). Church-based informal support
       among elderly blacks. The Gerontologist, 26(6), 637-642.

Frequency of church attendance in this sample is the most important predictor of frequency and amount of support. The most prevalent form of aid reported by these subjects was socioemotional support during illness.

Films

321   Clement, C. (Producer). (1979). Luna tune. WMM.

Luna Tune presents a sand animation of women's spirituality, with 80-year-old lesbian poet Elsa Gidlow reading her work, "What If...the Million and First Meditation."

Dissertations

322   Yeck, M. (1985). Effect of career status on the retirement needs of women religious. Unpublished doctoral dissertation, Michigan State University, 230p.

The researcher looks at the relationship between retirement needs of women religious and their differing career patterns. No significant relationship is found between career pattern and the intensity of response of the women religious, but occupational status forms a significant relationship with the need intensity of the respondents.

Housing

Books

323   Birch, E. (Ed.). (1985). Unsheltered woman: women and housing in the 80s. New Brunswick, New Jersey: Rutgers, The State University, Center for Urban Policy Research, 313p.

This collection of essays on defining gender-related needs, planning responsive projects and programs, and designing implementation strategies, presents a comprehensive view of housing analysis directed to women. Essays on demographic characteristics of the elderly in New York City and the Lenox Hill Neighborhood Association are especially relevant on the topic of women and aging.

Articles

324   Carp, F., & Christensen, D. (1986). Older women living alone: technical environmental assessment of psychological well-being. Research on Aging, 8(3), 407-435.

This article reports observation of effects of environmental measures and satisfaction with home and neighborhood on psychological well-being of older women.

325   Eckert, J., & Haug, M. (1984). The impact of forced residential relocation on the health of the elderly hotel dweller. The Journal of Gerontology, 39(6), 753-755.

Objective of this research is to assess the impact of involuntary relocation from one community setting to another on the self-perceived physical, functional, and emotional health status of older persons living in urban residential hotels. In general, there were few adverse changes in health associated with relocation among these subjects.

326 Fengler, A., & Danigelis, N. (1982). Residence, the elderly widow, and life satisfaction. Research on Aging, 4(1), 113-135.

Urban and rural widows are almost equally disadvantaged in objective ways, but urban widows perceive themselves to be considerably more disadvantaged than rural widows. The more urban the residence of the widow living alone, the lower her life satisfaction. All rural and urban widows living with children have higher life satisfaction than urban widows who live alone.

327 Hartwigsen, G. (1984-85). The appeal of the life care facility to the older widow. Journal of Housing for the Elderly, 2(4), 63-75.

Older widows are interviewed about relocation to a life care facility. Their primary reasons for moving are medical care, financial security, and safety. Their needs appear to have been met by the facility.

328 Harel, Z., Jackson, M., Deimling, G., & Noelker, L. (1983). Racial differences and well-being among aged and disabled public housing residents. Journal of Housing for the Elderly, 1(1), 45-62.

This examination of racial differences in well-being among aged and disabled public housing residents, predominantly female and widowed, suggests "the development and encouragement of mutual attention and assistance networks should be an important part of the organized effort to provide older persons with a living situation which is conducive to their helping themselves and each other as much as possible."

329 Hinrichsen, G. (1985). The impact of age-concentrated, publicly assisted housing on older people's social and emotional well-being. The Journal of Gerontology, 40(6), 758-760.

Living in age-concentrated housing, particularly high density senior citizen housing, is associated with "large numbers of friends, more active friendships, and slightly better morale but not with distinctive qualitative or structural aspects of social networks."

330 Hochschild, A. (1980). Communal life-styles for the old. In Fuller, M., & Martin, C. (Eds.), The older woman, pp. 289-303. Springfield, Illinois: Charles C Thomas, Publisher, 343p.

This case study of a small apartment building near San Francisco Bay of mainly conservative, fundamentalist widows, describes the development of feeling of community and bonding among residents of Merrill Court.

331 LaCayo, C. (1987). Inner city elderly. In Maddox, G. (Ed.), The encyclopedia of aging, pp. 353-355. New York: Springer Publishing Company, 890p.

Reports that central-city dwellers, increasingly, are poor, female, and members of minority groups. Compared to those in nonmetropolitan areas, there are significantly more women than men, and 46% of inner-city women are aged 65 and over. "Most older women and minorities are poor, so the proportion of poor inner-city seniors can be expected to increase."

332   Lally, M., Black, E., Thornock, M., & Hawkinds, J. (1980). Older
       women in single room occupant (SRO) hotels: a Seattle profile. In
       Fuller, M., & Martin, C. (Eds.), The older woman, pp. 304-316.
       Springfield, Illinois: Charles C. Thomas, Publisher, 343p.

Data collected from 16 older women living in ten hotels in downtown Seattle show a
strong value placed on independence, privacy, and autonomy, along with apparently limited
social networks.

333   McAuley, W., & Offerle, J. (1983). Perceived suitability of residence
       and life satisfaction among the elderly and handicapped. Journal of
       Housing for the Elderly, 1(1), 63-75.

The researchers look at those resources which influence the extent of social and physical
environments and whether the extensiveness of social and physical environments affect the
relationship between perceived residential suitability and life satisfaction. Most of the
sample are white, female, living alone, and with very low income.

334   Soldo, B., Sharma, M., & Campbell, R. (1984). Determinants of the
       community living arrangements of older unmarried women. Journal of
       Gerontology, 39(4), 492-498.

This study of older unmarried white women indicates that an unimpaired older woman has
a greater chance of living alone than an older woman who requires frequent assistance.
Women with the lowest incomes had less likelihood of living alone than those with higher
incomes.

Films

335   ACTION. (No date). There is no place like home.

These are stories of Senior Companions--men and women volunteers, 60 or older, who help
senior citizens "maintain their independence and continue to live in their own homes."

336   Martineau, B. (1982). Tales of tomorrow: our elders.

Helen has Alzheimer's disease; Sara, 80, a labor organizer and wheelchair activist, is
determined to live alone as long as she can. Both their stories are told.

337   McGraw-Hill Films. (1971). Nell and Fred.

Nell, 81, and Fred, 90, investigate moving into a new senior citizens' home in Montreal.

338   NFBC. (1956). The yellow leaf.

An elderly widow who moves into a home for the aged adjusts when she finds "congenial
friends, new interests, and a measure of independence."

339   Phoenix Films. (No date). Two worlds to remember.

Two elderly women adjust to moving to a home for the aged.

340   Pyramid. (1972). Tomorrow again.

A lonely older woman in an ancient resident hotel "desperately plans to seduce the attentions of the other guests by impressing them with her fur stole." After much preparation, she is not noticed, because other guests are too involved with themselves.

Documents

341   U.S. Congress. House. Subcommittee on Housing and Consumer Interests of the Select Committee on Aging. 98th Congress. (1984). Housing the elderly: alternative options (Erie, Pennsylvania), 51p.

The hearing considers housing concerns of older persons, with some examples given of situations of older women.

Dissertations

342   Abe-Ridder, L. (1983). The relationship of marital quality with sexual behavior and interest, morale, and sex role orientation for older couples living in two residential environments. Unpublished doctoral dissertation, The Florida State University, 334p.

Four hundred and eighty-eight males and females, 60 and over, married, and widowed, are studied on marital quality. Marital quality is not related to residential location (retirement community or in the community-at-large). Subjects claiming the highest quality marriages are significantly more likely to be sexually active and to report the highest frequencies of intercourse. Marital quality is not related to sex role orientation.

343   Gagnier, D. (1984). A comparative study of characteristics of management and elderly residents in homes for the aged in Michigan. Unpublished doctoral dissertation, The University of Michigan, 421p.

A state-wide survey of residential care facilities for the elderly, known as "homes for the aged" in Michigan, compares management characteristics and elderly residents.

344   Hunn, D. (1984). A plan that failed: a solar retirement housing development in Marin County, California. Unpublished doctoral dissertation, Claremont Graduate School, 133p.

This research describes the development and failure of a 280-unit model solar energy retirement community in California.

345   Miller, E.   (1985).   Elderly females living alone: an ethnographic
      study.   Unpublished   doctoral   dissertation,   Columbia   University
      Teachers College, 261p.

From November 1982 to August 1984, three elderly female informants were studied.
Inferences were that elderly females can learn, more slowly than younger, but in different
areas of life; that successful social mediative influences can create the appropriate
conditions for successful learning; that, through religion, the elderly female fulfills social
functions to satisfy her need for belongingness and recognition.

346   Schreter, C.   (1983).   Rooms for rent: shared housing with nonrelated
      older Americans.   Unpublished   doctoral   dissertation,   Bryn   Mawr
      College, 222p.

This research compares private sector, self-initiated home-sharers to clients of a housemate-
matching service and to group household members living in agency-sponsored group
homes.   The researcher concludes that shared housing, if including self-initiated, agency-
assisted, and agency-sponsored shared householders, appears to be an intergenerational and
flexible living arrangement which serves as economic, social, or physical needs of people in
transition.

347   Story, B.   (1983).   A comparison of self-esteem of older adults in age-
      segregated and age-integrated residential environments.   Unpublished
      doctoral dissertation, The Ohio State University, 150p.

One hundred and twenty older adults, including 86 females, are compared on self-esteem,
based on different living environments.   Characteristics of age-integrated residential
environment may be conducive to the positive self-esteem of older adults.   Individuals who
perceive themselves to have good health are more inclined to have a positive outlook than
individuals who perceive themselves as being in poor health.

348   Wyckoff, S.   (1983).   The effects of housing and race upon depression
      and life satisfaction of elderly females.   Unpublished doctoral
      dissertation, George Peabody College for Teachers of Vanderbilt
      University, 143p.

One hundred and forty-four black and white females, 65 and older, are subjects in this
study.   There is no significant difference between these subjects in planned and unplanned
housing with regard to depression and life satisfaction.   White females in planned housing
showed a higher level of life satisfaction than black females who resided in planned
housing.   Black females in unplanned housing reported a lower level of depression than
white females residing in unplanned housing.

Racial and Ethnic Groups

Books

349   Becerra, R., & Shaw, D. (1984). The Hispanic elderly: a research reference guide. Lanham, Maryland: University Press of America, 144p.

This guide to Spanish-language research instruments describes instruments which have been, or are now being, used to assess the Hispanic elderly.

350   Driedger, L., and Chappell, N. (1987). Aging and ethnicity: toward an interface. Toronto: Butterworths, 131p.

The critique of research and policy literature on aging and ethnicity in Canada includes a short section on gender differentials.

351   Hayes, C., Kalish, R., and Guttman, D. (Eds.). (1986). European-American elderly: a guide for practice. New York: Springer Publishing Company, 272p.

Included in this collection are a demographic profile of older Euro-Americans, family assistance, and programs and services for the Euro-American elderly.

352   Johnson, C. (1985). Growing up and growing old in Italian-American families. New Brunswick, New Jersey: Rutgers University Press, 245p.

Italian-Americans' views on marriage, education, parental care, social mobility, women's roles are analyzed. Interdependence among generations is the norm. For economic reasons, many Italian-American women work to supplement the family income and cannot take care of elderly parents on a regular basis.

353   Manuel, R. (Ed.). (1982). Minority aging: sociological and social
       psychological issues. Westport, Connecticut: Greenwood Press, 285p.

These essays on the lifelong socialization of the minority experience describe the lifestyle
of the minority aged and ways used by the minority aged to cope successfully with
problems.

354   Markides, K., & Martin, H., with the assistance of Gomez, E. (1983).
       Older Mexican Americans: a study in an urban barrio. Austin, Texas:
       The Center for Mexican American Studies, The University of Texas,
       139p.

The book covers socioeconomic characteristics, family structure and family relations,
psychological well-being, health status and health care utilization, religious behavior, and
retirement patterns of Mexican Americans.

355   McNeely, R., & Cohen, J. (Eds.). (1983). Aging in minority groups.
       Beverly Hills: Sage Publications, 300p.

These papers focus on differences among and within subpopulations of the aged. Included
are Asian-Pacific elderly, Mexican-Americans, Blacks, Cubans, and Native Americans.

Articles/chapters

356   Bastida, E. (1984). Reconstructing the social world at 60:   older
       Cubans in the United States. Gerontologist, 24(5), 465-470.

The article examines older Cubans who live in Miami, Florida, with regard to their
creativity in using resources.

357   Chatters, L., Taylor, R., & Jackson, J. (1985). Size and composition
       of the informal helper networks of elderly Blacks. Journal of
       Gerontology, 40(5), 605-614.

This study focuses on the relationship among sociodemographic, health, family, and
availability factors to the size and composition of the informal support network. "The
findings underscore the importance of availability and family factors in support
relationships and the relative ineffectiveness of health factors as predictors of network size
and composition."

358   Cohler, B., Lieberman, M. (1980). Social relations and mental health:
       middle-aged and older men and women from three European ethnic
       groups. Research on Aging, 1(4), 445-469.

Irish, Italian, and Polish subjects were measured on the nature and extent of social ties, life-
event stress, and positive morale and psychological impairment. Among Italian and Polish
women in (the two most "socially bonded" groups), "increased involvement with significant
others was associated both with increased life stress and less than satisfactory personal
adjustment."

359   Conway, K. (1985-86). Coping with the stress of medical problems
       among black and white elderly. International Journal of Aging and
       Human Development, 21(1), 39-48.

Coping responses of a group of low-income black and white urban elderly women to the
stressful event of a medical problem are investigated. The black elderly engaged in social
support, prayer, and nonprescription drugs more frequently.

360   Dilworth-Anderson, P.   (1984).   A sociological overview of older
       minority women. In Bastida, E. (Ed.), Older women: current issues
       and problems, pp. 56-67, Volume 2 of Convergence in Aging. Kansas
       City, Kansas: Mid-America Congress on Aging, 136p.

Compares older minority women in America to older white women with regard to
education, job discrimination, and family ties.   Four ethnic groups included are Asians,
blacks, Native Americans, and Hispanics.

361   Edwards, E.   (1983).   Native-American elders: current issues and
       social policy implications. In McNeely, R., & Cohen, J. (Eds.), Aging
       in minority groups, pp. 74-84. Beverly Hills: Sage Publications.

Looks at economics, health, mental health, housing, family support of Native American
elders.   Over half of Indian women 60 and over are widowed and have problems of
loneliness, inadequate transportation, and lack of resources for home maintenance and
family support systems.

362   Gelfand, D.   (1986).   Families, assistance, and the Euro-American
       elderly. In Hayes, C. L., Kalish, R. A., Guttman, D. (Eds.), European-
       American elderly: a guide for practice, pp 79-93.   New York:
       Springer Publishing Company, 272p.

Includes section on women's roles and obligations within the family unit.

363   Greene, V., & Monahan, D.   (1984).   Comparative utilization of
       community based long term care services by Hispanic and Anglo
       elderly in a case management system. Journal of Gerontology, 39(6),
       730-735.

Comparison of use of formal and informal supports by Hispanic and Anglo elderly.
Hispanic elderly, in general, used significantly fewer agency services than did Anglo
elderly, although Hispanics showed greater impairment. Hispanic elderly used significantly
higher levels of informal support.

364   Hayes, C.   (1986).   Resources and services benefiting the Euro-
       American elderly.   In Hayes, C. L., Kalish, R. A., & Guttman, D.
       (Eds.), European-American elderly: a guide for practice, pp. 180-197.
       New York: Springer Publishing Company, 272p.

Includes discussion of ethnic women's attitudes toward aging, role models, and coping with
caregiving.

365   Holloway, K., & Demetrakopoulos, S.   (1986).   Remembering our
       foremothers: older black women, politics of age, politics of survival as
       embodied in the novels of Toni Morrison. In Bell, M. J. (Ed.), Women
       as elders: images, visions, and issues, pp. 13-34.   New York:
       Harrington Press, 90p.

Novelist Toni Morrison's works are described in terms of American culture, literary
originality, Black feminism, and women's spirituality. The authors conclude that Black
culture, based on an African ethos, values the feminine and the aged so much more than
white culture does.

366   Johnson, E. (1981-82). Role expectations and role realities of older
       Italian mothers and their daughters. International Journal of Aging
       and Human Development, 14(4), 271-276.

Ninety pairs of Italian-Americans, single, older women and their daughters, were studied.
The quality of relationships was perceived as quite high and there was high consensus for
the expectations and realities of the role responsibilities of parents and children. Mothers
showed more role confusion about what they felt children should expect and what they
themselves could provide. Daughters may desire less advice and more emotional support
from their mothers.

367   Kiefer, C., Kim, S., Choi, K., Kim, L., Kim, B.-L., Shon, S., & Kim, T.
       (1985).   Adjustment problems of Korean American elderly.
       Gerontologist, 25(5), 477-482.

Interviews with 50 elderly Korean immigrants to identify typical adjustment problems of
this group. Adjustment was found to be positively related to education, length of residence
in the United States, and multigenerational household structure.

368   Lee, C-F. (1986). A demographic profile of older Euro-Americans.
       In Hayes, C. L., Kalish, R. A., & Guttman, D.   (Eds.), European-
       American elderly: a guide for practice, pp. 51-76.   New York:
       Springer Publishing Company, 272p.

Euro-American immigrants are overrepresented among old and old-old, largely because the
flow of immigrants from Europe has declined since the early decades of this century.
Women substantially outnumber men and most of these women are widowed. Census data
and data from New York City are cited.

369   Liang, J., Van Tran, T., & Markides, K. (1988). Differences in the
       structure of life satisfaction index in three generations of Mexican
       Americans. Journal of Gerontology: Social Sciences, 43, S1-8.

Study investigates differences in the structure of seven Life Satisfaction Index items across
three generations of Mexican Americans.   About two-thirds of the subjects in each
generation were women.

370   Manton, K. (1982). Differential life expectancy: possible explanations
        during the later ages. In Manuel, R. C.   (Ed.), Minority aging:
        sociological and psychological issues, pp. 63-68. Westport, Connecticut:
        Greenwood Press.

Females, within one race, tend to have a greater life expectancy, higher probability of
survival at age X, and lower probability of death at age X.   Nonwhite males and females
begin life with a considerable mortality disadvantage on all three indices.   At more
advanced ages, these individuals become advantaged.

371   Manuel, R., & Reid, J.   (1982).   A comparative demographic profile of
        the minority and nonminority aged. In Manuel, R. C.   (Ed.), Minority
        aging: sociological and social psychological issues, pp. 31-52.
        Westport, Connecticut: Greenwood Press.

Demographic data indicate that there are more females, increasing by age category, within
each ethnic category.

372   Markides, K., & Vernon, S.   (1984).   Aging, sex-role orientation, and
        adjustment: a three-generations study of Mexican Americans. Journal
        of Gerontology, 39(5), 586-591.

This article investigates the hypothesis that "less traditional sex-role orientation is positively
related to psychological well-being and that this relationship is stronger among the older
than among younger generations."   Traditional sex-role orientation was found to be
positively related to depression among older women and to depression and life satisfaction
in younger males.   Traditional sex-role orientation was not related to well-being in older
males.

373   Markides, K., Boldt, J., & Ray, L.   (1986).   Sources of helping and
        intergenerational solidarity: a three-generation study of Mexican-
        Americans. Journal of Gerontology, 41(4), 506-511.

The authors examine sources of help and advice (other than from one's spouse) and the
extent of solidarity among generations among three generations of Mexican-Americans.   In
all generations studied, the family was predominantly the source of support.   "Women are
relied on for help regarding health matters and men regarding home repairs and upkeep.
Help and advice regarding financial problems and personal problems fall primarily along
same-sex lines.   Scales measuring intergenerational solidarity showed that all-female dyads
have greater associational solidarity than all-male and cross-sex dyads.

374   McNeely, R.   (1983).   Race, sex, and victimization of the elderly.   In
        McNeely, R. L., & Cohen, J. H.   (Eds.), Aging in minority groups, pp.
        137-152. Beverly Hills: Sage Publications.

Data used in this study were the National Crime Survey analysis. of victimization rates
(personal victimizations include any offenses involving face-to-face confrontation or victim
offender contact by race and gender).   Although they were victimized less often than
others, the threat of potential victimization and its consequences are of great concern to
elders--especially for elderly women living alone who tended to be in the poorest financial
situations.   Older minority women were found to have the highest exposure to risk of
personal victimization of all aged subgroups.

375   Miller, J. (1984). Older black women as workers. In Women, work, and age: policy challenge. Ann Arbor: Institute of Gerontology, University of Michigan, 26p.

Four themes emerged in this study: "invisibility of the older black woman worker, the historical and future trends that affect the older black woman of today and of tomorrow, the special circumstances--in needs, experiences, and problem-solving--that must be considered when discussing older black women as workers, and the inappropriateness of programs designed for white men and women and black men, but applied to older black women."

376   Ralston, P. (1984). Senior center utilization by black elderly adults: social, attitudinal, and knowledge correlates. Journal of Gerontology, 39(2), 224-229.

An examination of factors affecting use of senior centers by black elderly adults. Gender did not have a significant effect on any of the variables studied.

377   Rao, V., & Rao, V. (1981-82). Life satisfaction in the black elderly: an exploratory study. International Journal of Aging and Human Development, 14(1), 55-65.

In this study, 240 black elderly, 59% females, were included. However, gender results were not given. The Life Satisfaction Index-A was used.

378   Snyder, P. (1984). Health service implications of folk healing among older Asian Americans and Hawaiians in Honolulu. Gerontologist, 24(5), 471-476.

There were more older women than men among this group of Asian and Hawaiian healers. The women generally had made substantial contributions to their families' well-being, but wage-earning was not their primary activity. The healers received high monetary rewards, but "healers are not expected to become wealthy from such work. Some felt marriage and healing were not compatible because of the demands by clients on a healer's time and the intense personal involvement of the healer in the process."

379   Spurlock, J. (1984). Black women in the middle years. In Baruch, G., & Brooks-Gunn, J. (Eds.), Women in midlife, pp. 245-260. New York: Plenum Press, 404p.

For a great percentage of black women, they are likely to age quickly and are vulnerable to disorders related to poverty. The overwhelming majority of black women arrive, in their middle years, burdened by economic problems. Emphasis was placed on the diversity among black women--"...what is brought to middle age depends upon how life has dealt with us before and how we have dealt with life."

380   Taylor, R. (1985). The extended family as a source of support to elderly blacks. Gerontologist, 25(5), 488-495.

There were 581 blacks, 55 and over, in this study. Income, education, region, degree of family interaction, proximity of relatives, and having adult children were found to be determinants of frequency of support.

381   Taylor, S. (1982). **Mental health and successful coping among aged Black women.** In Manuel, R. C. (Ed.), <u>Minority aging: sociological and psychological issues,</u> pp. 95-100.   Westport, Connecticut: Greenwood Press.

The sample of elderly black women, 59-97, was from a metropolitan New England community. "Values emphasizing faith, family, and a strong adherence to the American work ethic shape coping strategies and allow individuals to use kinship connections as problem-solving devices.   Belief in family support (whether family is supportive or negligent) is the primary strategy letting older women define aging as no big thing."

382   Usui, W. (1984). **Homogeneity of friendship networks of elderly blacks and whites.** <u>Journal of Gerontology,</u> 29(3), 350-356.

Examines friendship networks of elderly males and females with regard to race, sex, age, marital status, and education. Women were found to have greater sex homogeneity in friendships--i.e., men tended to have more cross-sex friendships than did women.

383   Wolf, J., Breslau, N., Ford, A., Ziegler, H., & Ward, A.   (1983). **Distance and contacts: interactions of black urban elderly adults with family and friends.** <u>Journal of Gerontology,</u> 38(4), 465-471.

Contacts with family and friends of 655 black urban residents 60 and older were investigated. The neighborhood was found to be an important place for socializing with family and friends (also the case for working-class white elderly adults). "Social contacts increase with higher income for working-class elderly whites; for these black working-class and poor elderly adults, social contacts decrease with higher income."

384   Yu, L., & Wu, S-C. (1985). **Unemployment and family dynamics in meeting the needs of Chinese elderly in the United States.** <u>Gerontologist,</u> 25(5), 472-476.

A study of effects of unemployment on the discomfort level of providing financial support and housing for a group of Midwestern Chinese-American elderly. One spouse's discomfort in meeting the needs of elderly relatives affected the other spouse's discomfort.   The married, employed females were most likely to give money to parents and in-laws. Employment was found to decrease the discomfort level of respondents who were helping older relatives.

Films

385   Almond, P. (Producer). (1980). <u>A private life.</u>

Two aging German-Jewish immigrants in New York City try to find love and companionship as they adjust to aging and dislocation.

386   Ashur, G. (1977). Me and Stella: a film about Elizabeth Cotton.

An elderly black woman, amateur guitarist, singer, and songwriter who gained recognition in her later years and her guitar named Stella are the foci of this film. He story proves that neither age nor race need impede in the world of folk music.

387   Burdeau, G. (1976). A season of grandmothers.

Emphasis is on the role of the grandmother in American Indian life, with examples from Spokane, Coeur d'Alene, and Nez Perce tribes, Kootenai, Flathead, Kalispel reservation, and Colville.

388   Knight, C. (Producer). (1974). Old, black and alive!

The film presents six elderly blacks living in Macon County, Alabama, and depicts their daily lives there.

389   Learning Corporation of America. (1973). Autobiography of Miss Jane Pittman.

The biography of black former slave Jane Pittman covers a period from post-Civil War time to a civil rights march 100 years later.

390   Marton, D. (Producer). Dona Maria. (1981). (Also video).

A 100-year-old Mexican curandera (healer), explains her philosophy and her traditional healing methods.

391   McGannon, J. (No date). 56 1/2 Howard Street.

Marguerite Osborn, 84, of Indian and Black ancestry, has been harassed in her neighborhood, but shows enthusiasm and spirit in dealing with her situation.

392   Newberry Award Records. (Producer). (1979). Annie and the old one. (Disc or cassette).

In this film, Annie, a Navajo girl, learns about living and dying from her wise grandmother.

393   Nunez, V. (Producer). (1973). Taking care of Mother Baldwin.

This story describes the strained relations between an older black woman and her young, teen-aged handyman in the rural South.

394   NYF (Producer). (1953). Tokyo Story. (Japanese/subtitled).

An elderly couple's journey to Tokyo results in a "less than warm" welcome by their children. Generational conflicts are set aside, temporarily, by death.

395   Obomsawin, A. (Producer). (1978). Mother of many children.

The memories of Agatha Marie Goodine, 108, a member of the Hobbema tribe, are contrasted with the conflicts faced by many Indian and Inuit women today.

396   Parsons, J. (Producer). (1981). Luisa Torres (within America). (Video).

This documentary reveals one day in the family life of a 79-year-old woman, from her gathering of herbs to washing a mattress to selecting the tree from which her casket will be made.

397   Patrick, S. (produced 1975, released 1982). A thousand moons.

"More than a thousand moons have come and gone since the birth of Regina, a mixed blood matriarch now living in the big city poverty where she senses that death is imminent. She knows she must return to her distant birthplace to be welcomed by the spirits of her Indian ancestors." The film shows her son and his friends trying to make her wish come true.

398   Pyramid Films. (1973). Legend days are over.

Modern society's intrusions into the life of the Indian people are lamented by an old Indian woman.

399   Sternberg, T., Wang, W., Yung, D., & Tai, V. (1986). Dim sum: a little bit of heart.

Mrs. Tam, in her early sixties, begins to prepare for death, but experiences a spiritual rebirth. Intergenerational relations with her daughter are also emphasized.

400   Teleketics. (1975). With just a little trust.

An elderly black woman, feet swollen with arthritis, travels through an urban ghetto to help her daughter, widowed and with three children.

401   WNET (Producer). (1972). Rose Argoff.

The story of Rose Argoff illustrates what it is like to be old, poor, and Jewish on the lower East Side of New York City.

Documents

402   Report of the Mini-Conference on Pacific/Asian Elderly.   (No date). Pacific/Asians: the wisdom of age, 11p.

The 1981 White House Conference on Aging document prepared for consideration of the Conference delegates, along with recommendations.

403   U.S. Congress. House. Congressional Black Caucus, "Brain Trust on Aging," and the Select Committee on Aging. 99th Congress. (1986). The black elderly in poverty, 68p.

"Health care rationing" already in effect--according to Social Security Administration, 69 percent of all older single black women had incomes at 125% of poverty level in 1982; thus, their income renders them ineligible for Medicaid. Presents an overview of the black poor elderly: income maintenance, health care and health care costs, Social Security.

404   U.S. Congress. House. Select Committee on Aging. 99th Congress. (1986). Health care problems of the black aged, 116p.

Report of hearing held to highlight continuing health needs of black elderly persons in the United States. Includes brief press release from Central Detroit Older Women's League, citing 89% of all black women, 55 years and older, who live at poverty line, have no health insurance and 60% of all black females, age 40 and over, have limited pension and retirement benefits, and as they age their health care benefits deteriorate.

405   U.S. Congress. House.   Select Committee on Aging. 98th Congress. (1984). Minority elderly and low-income needs: New York, 65p.

Examples of older minority women included in this hearing report.   Topics include: housing, income, nutrition, health care, cultural differences, handicapping conditions, Blacks, Hispanics, Puerto Ricans.

Dissertations

406   Artean, D. (1982). Rural elderly Mexican-Americans: an assessment of functioning in daily living.   Unpublished doctoral dissertation, University of Maryland, 125p.

Investigates factors influencing the social, psychological, and physical functioning of rural elderly Mexican-Americans in three counties in West Texas. No significant differences in cumulative impairment ratings by sex found.

407   Barber, J. (1983). Old age and the life course of slaves: a case study of a nineteenth century Virginia plantation.   Unpublished doctoral dissertation, University of Kansas, 447p.

Studies the life course of 577 American slaves, focusing on old age. "Older workers were generally devalued, even when they occupied positions of occupational authority." "Retirement" was more common among women than among men and was probably related to declining health.

408   Capozzoli, M. (1985). **Three generations of Italian American women in Nassau County, New York, 1925-1981.** Unpublished doctoral dissertation, Lehigh University, 300p.

Interviews, questionnaires, censuses, and historical sources were used to examine women's work, education, religion, sexual morality, and household and leisure activities. "Being Italian was important in the lives of these women."

409   Connors, D. (1986). **"I've always had everything I've wanted--but I never wanted very much": an experiential analysis of Irish-American working class women in their nineties.** Unpublished doctoral dissertation, Brandeis University, 198p.

Study of the lives of sex New England women in their nineties of working-class, Irish-descent. Focus on the survival strategies they developed.

410   Irvin, Y. (1982). **The relationship of age and adjustment to the subjective well-being of older black women.** Unpublished doctoral dissertation, University of Pittsburgh, 12p.

Investigation of the relationship between age, observed adjustment, and subjective well-being in young-old (60-75) and old-old (76+) black women participants in multiservice daycare programs.

411   Koh, Y. (1983). **An exploratory study of filial support and the use of formal services among the Korean aged in New York City.** Unpublished doctoral dissertation, The Florida State University, 258p.

Sample of Korean elderly in the New York City area who migrated to the United States within the past decade. Focus of this research was on living arrangements of Korean elders, pattern of help between children and aging parents, and the use of formal services by Korean elderly.

412   Lewis, V. (1983). **The mid-life concerns of minority women returning to school during middle age: a developmental perspective.** Unpublished doctoral dissertation, Wayne State University, 137p.

Research on the extent to which the mid-life crisis occurs in the life minority women returning to school and whether they have specific development concerns. Findings were that minority women experience introspective concerns (focus on one's mental and emotional state) and concerns about role as wife.

413   Litwin-Grinberg, R. (1982). **Lives in retrospect: a qualitative analysis of oral reminiscence as applied to elderly Jewish women.** Unpublished doctoral dissertation,, University of California, Berkeley, 204p.

Eight Jewish women, 76 to 92, born in Eastern Europe, emigrants to the United States, tended to reevaluate their lives through a conscious search for the meaning of important events and experiences.

414   Meyer, S. (1986). **An investigation of self-concept change in black re-entry women.** Unpublished doctoral dissertation, Columbia University Teachers College, 228p.

Investigates the experiences of Black women enrolled in college after a lengthy absence from formal education. Positive self-concept found as result of college attendance and of entering the work force.

415   Phillips, G. (1983). **The quality of life among Black and Hispanic elderly in three southern cities.** Unpublished doctoral dissertation, University of Pennsylvania, 313p.

An existing data set from the four-year national evaluation of the Community Development Black Grant Program was used. Findings were that objective and subjective indicators are influential in determining the quality of life experiences among racial-ethnic minority elderly in the South.

416   Powers, M. (1982). **Oglala women in myth, ritual, and reality.** Unpublished doctoral dissertation, Rutgers University The State University of New Jersey (Ne Brunswick), 347p.

Study of relationship between sex roles and social structure and extent to which contemporary female leaders model their own lives after what they perceive to be traditional Indian roles. Twenty years of interviews with females aged 16 to 96 are included.

417   Sanchez-Ayendez, M. (1984). **Puerto Rican elderly women: aging in an ethnic minority group in the United States.** Unpublished doctoral dissertation, University of Massachusetts, 333p.

Cultural value orientations are seen as central to understanding how minority elders approach growing old and how they meet the changes associated with aging. Description of values and behavior in the social networks and daily lives of older Puerto Rican women and the cultural continuities that structure the process of aging for them.

418   Taylor, R. (1983). **The informal social support networks of the black elderly: the impact of family, church members, and best friends.** Unpublished doctoral dissertation, The University of Michigan, 356p.

Elderly Black females were more likely to receive family support than males. Subjects in this study were most likely to receive total and instrumental support from their families, companionship from their friends, and advice, encouragement, or help during sickness from church members.

419   Terry, R. (1982). <u>Diet, anthropometric characteristics, and diabetes-related attitudes and knowledge among women residing in the Eastern Cherokee township of Snowbird.</u> Unpublished doctoral dissertation, The University of Tennessee, 180p.

Census of 105 Snowbird women, ages 18 to 87. Older women and women in the upper Indian inheritance quartile had a greater prevalence of previously diagnosed diabetes.

Policy Issues

Books

420   Giele, J. (Ed.).   (1982).   **Women in the middle years: current knowledge and directions for research and policy.**   New York: John Wiley & Sons, 283p.

This book gives a cross-disciplinary perspective of the challenges and crises facing the midlife woman. Women's middle years are viewed by experts from medicine, psychology, psychiatry, anthropology, and sociology.   Includes contributions on adult women, biomedical data, marriage, work and family roles, women in the German Democratic Republic, and future policy and research questions.   Concludes with appendix describing longitudinal and cross-sectional data sources on women in the middle years.

421   King, N., & Marvel, M.   (1982).   **Issues, policies, and programs for midlife and older women.**   Washington, D.C.:   Center for Women Policy Studies, 166p.

This is a report and analysis of a national survey of programs for midlife and older women.

422   Michigan, University of.   (1984).   **Women, work, and age: policy challenge.**   Ann Arbor: Institute of Gerontology, University of Michigan, 26p.

This describes proceedings of a conference sponsored by a Michigan coalition of educational and research institutions, government agencies, and advocacy organizations. Workshop reports on organizing financial security, age and sex discrimination in the workplace, employment and training opportunities, life planning.   Keynote address included on the invisible barriers of age discrimination.

423   Szinovacz, M.   (Ed.)   (1982).   **Women's retirement: policy implications of recent research.** Beverly Hills: Sage Publications, 271p.

This collection of research focuses on women's retirement. Emphasis is on the impact of work history and employment status on the life situation of the older woman, attitudes toward retirement and retirement preparation, and the determinants and consequences of retirement for women. The bibliography includes "most of the publications on women's retirement published within the last decade."

Articles/chapters

424   Cutler, S. (1983). **Aging and changes in attitudes about the women's liberation movement. International Journal of Aging and Human Development, 16**(1), 43-51.

The author uses data from a four-year national panel study, examining changes in attitudinal support from the women's liberation movement 1972-1976. All age groups became more favorable (toward the movement), but the extent of these shifts was greater among the older members of the panel than among the younger members. There was no support for the idea that social and political attitudes became more conservative with aging or that they became rigid and fixed.

425   Hess, B. (1986). **Antidiscrimination policies today and the life chances of older women tomorrow. The Gerontologist, 26**, 132-135.

If existing statutes are not enforced and there continue to be structural changes in the economy, "women's economic disadvantages in the workplace will continue through this century, despite increased educational attainment and labor force participation. This is especially true for women of color and Hispanic origin, but all women run the risk of outliving their resources. Proposed remedies such as earnings sharing and pay equity have received the support from the current administration."

426   Markson, E. (1987). **Older women's movement.** In Maddox, G. (Ed.), **The encyclopedia of aging,** pp. 502-504. New York: Springer Publishing Company, 890p.

Specific organizations focusing on women in the second half of life have developed relatively recently in the twentieth century, during the early 1970s. Proportionately few older women are members of the Older Women's League or other similar organizations advancing the interests of women in late life.

Films

427   CBS News (Producer). (1981). **Thoroughly modern Millicent.**

This films provides a profile of Millicent Fenwick [then] congressional representative from New Jersey. Elected for the first time at age 64, she is direct, "dead-honest," the "conscience of the Congress."

428   IU (1975). Maggie Kuhn: wrinkled radical.

Sixty-nine-year-old Maggie Kuhn, organizer of the Gray Panthers, is interviewed by author Studs Terkel.

429   Michigan, University of, Institute of Gerontology.   (1979).   Portrait: Maggie Kuhn.

Maggie Kuhn, national convenor of the Gray Panther network, is interviewed on projects, issues, achievements, and aspirations of the Gray Panthers, and "her hopes for younger Americans."

Documents

430   Block, M., Davidson, J., & Gelfand, D.   (1983).   Working paper 1: policy framework handbook. College Park, Maryland: National Policy Center on Women and Aging, 91p.

This document covers global issues, circumscribed sex roles, acute responsive health care system, 1980 census data analysis.   Major issues affecting older women, outcomes stemming from these issues, and policy options for altering the condition of older women on these issues are discussed. Global issues discussed include limited occupational choice, disparity between male-female earnings, high unemployment, high volunteerism, misfit of employment patterns with retirement income systems, high risk of poverty.

431   Cahn, A. (1979).   Midlife women: policy Proposals on their problems, 21p.

A summary of papers submitted to the Subcommittee on Retirement Income and Employment of the Select Committee on Aging of the U.S. House of Representatives, 96th Congress. Views of 29 experts on 18 topics affecting midlife women are presented. All authors are unanimous in stressing the importance of building a solid foundation in the middle years. Considered are such issues as midlife women's future, role changes, work and education, displaced homemakers, volunteer work, preparation for retirement, continuing education, work and family, psychological factors, new careers, pensions, poverty, counseling and guidance, mutual help, age discrimination, alternative housing, public office, and prospects.

432   Federal Council on the Aging. (1975).   National policy concerns for older women: commitment to a better life, 51p.

This document reports a 1975 public hearing by the Federal Council on the Aging of national policy concerns for older women.

433   New York (State) Legislature, Assembly, Task Force on Women's
       Issues and the Assembly Standing Committee on Aging. (1983). The
       status of older women, 18p.

This report summarizes four public hearings on the status of older women. Held in 1983
by the New York State Assembly Task Force on Women's Issues and the Standing
Committee on Aging to examine the unique problems facing women in their later years and
the lifelong circumstances that contribute to those problems. Recommendations included
exempting greater portion of estates from state and federal taxes to allow greater means of
support for widows and promoting programs in financial, estate, and retirement planning to
help women cope with widowhood and divorce.

434   U.S. Congress. Senate. Special Committee on Aging. 99th Congress.
       (1986). Challenges for women: taking charge, taking care, 79p.

The hearing proceedings examine aging of the population, especially changing roles of
women. Caregiving, grandparents' rights, housing needs, nutrition programs, medical care,
respite care are covered.

435   U.S. Congress. Senate. Special Committee on Aging. 98th Congress.
       (1984). Women in our aging society, 107p.

Health reform, Medicare and Social Security, pension reform, the gender gap in aging,
home health care, chronic health problems, long-term care insurance, age discrimination in
employment, poverty, pensions are included in this discussion.

Dissertations

436   Weiler, N. (1983). The aged, the family, and the problems of a
       maturing industrial society, New York, 1900-1930. Unpublished
       doctoral dissertation, University of Illinois at Chicago, 330p.

The changing reality of life for older persons and the development of public policy during
an important time of change are analyzed. "Interest in the elderly arose after the economy
was already industrialized, but before social welfare schemes had been worked out in the
United States." Sample is from New York state census of 1925, when 70% of those 65
and older lived with spouses and or children. As long as they remained married (60% of
men and 30% of women), most retained the status of household head regardless of age and
regardless of employment.

International Concerns

Books

437   American Association for International Aging. (1986). <u>Aging and the
       global agenda for women: conversations in Nairobi.</u>   Washington,
       D.C.: American Association for International Aging, 34p.

This report of the international dialogues on older women held at Forum '85, the
nongovernmental segment United Nations Conference for Women ending the United
Nations Decade for Women. Summarizes the workshops on older women and provides
suggestions for future action.

438   Datan, N., Antonovsky, A., & Mapz, B. (1981). <u>A time to reap: the
       middle age of women in five Israeli subcultures.</u> Baltimore: Johns
       Hopkins University Press, 194p.

Five groups who have made the normative transitions of the life cycle from youth to
maturity against a backdrop of geographical and cultural transitions--Central Europeans,
Turks, Persians, North Africans, Israel-born Moslem Arab women--are studied. "Women in
all five sub-cultures value the companionship of a good marriage and cherish their children,
while seeking personal autonomy and the satisfaction of a job well done."

439   Gibson, M. (1985). <u>Older women around the world.</u> Washington,
       D.C.: International Federation on Ageing, in cooperation with the
       American Association of Retired Persons, 58p.

This monograph provides an overview of older women's roles in the family, their income
and employment status, and their health care needs, and provides suggestions for steps to
be taken by governments and nongovernmental organizations. The focus is on encouraging
policymakers, planners, and service-providers to address the diverse needs of older women
in their societies.

440   Ikels, C. (1983). **Aging and adaptation: Chinese in Hong Kong and the United States.** Hamden, Connecticut: Archon Books, 262p.

The study of elderly Chinese emigrants to Hong Kong and greater Boston reveals how elderly men and women modify traditional solutions to minimize the hardship of being old in a new and strange environment.

441   Nusberg, C., & Sokolovsky, J. (Eds.). (1987). **The international directory of research and researchers in comparative gerontology.** The International Federation on Ageing, 196p.

Identifies key research projects with policy and program relevance, facilitating communication among researchers focusing on comparative gerontology. Lists and describes research projects.

442   Peace, S. (1981). **An international perspective on the status of older women.** Washington, D.C.: International Federation on Ageing, 92p.

This report for a presentation at the United Nations World Conference, "Decade for Women--Equality, Development and Peace" in July 1980 looks at the recommendations adopted by the World Conference in "International Women's Year" in 1975 which were focused on the needs and opportunities of young and middle-aged women, while the status of older women was "sadly neglected." The publication discusses roles and images, health, income issues, family-related roles, and presents a demographic and sociological profile of older women.

443   Raybeck, D. (1983). **Kelantan Malay and traditional Chinese perspectives on middle-aged women: a diminished dichotomy.** East Lansing, Michigan: Women in International Development, Michigan State University, 13p.

As women age, the status of both Kelantanese and Chinese women increases--the former because of extra-domestic activities and the latter because of alterations in the domestic situation.

Articles/chapters

444   Berg, S., Mellstrom, D., Persson, G., & Svanborg, A. (1981). Loneliness in the Swedish Aged. **Journal of Gerontology,** 36(3), 342-349.

Feelings of loneliness in relation to disease, handicaps, social network, and social background of 1,007 70-year-old people living in Sweden are studied. Loneliness is a problem to 24% of the women and to 12% of the men. The most important factors related to feeling lonely are loss of spouse, depression of mood, and lack of friends.

445   Campbell, R., & Brody, E. (1985). Women's changing roles and help to the elderly: attitudes of women in the United States and Japan. **Gerontologist,** 25(6), 584-592.

A three-generation study of women's attitudes toward gender-appropriate roles and filial responsibility shows more egalitarian gender-role attitudes in the United States than in Japan. In both the U.S. and Japan, all three generations agree that the family is responsible for care of the elderly, but Americans have more positive attitudes toward filial responsibility than do the Japanese.

446   Cohler, B. (1982). Stress or support: relations between older women
       from three European ethnic groups and their relatives. In Manuel, R.
       C. (Ed.), Minority aging: sociological and psychological issues, pp. 115-
       120. Westport, Connecticut: Greenwood Press.

Within ethnic communities such as Italian- and Polish-Americans, women are very important in maintaining interdependence among relatives on a continuing basis. Continuing ties among relatives may lessen strain among young adults, but among older adults, especially midlife women, continuing family ties "represent a source of decreased life satisfaction and are often experienced as the source rather than solution of strains associated with life in contemporary urban society."

447   Collette, J. (1984). Sex differences in life satisfaction: Australian
       data. Journal of Gerontology, 39(2), 243-245.

One thousand and fifty elderly males and females are analyzed for sex differences in life satisfaction and its determinants. There are few differences between sexes found in determining life satisfaction. There is little or no interaction between sex and the other variables examined.

448   Cruz-Lopez, M., & Pearson, R. (1985). The support needs and
       resources of Puerto Rican elders. Gerontologist, 25(5), 483-487.

Older Puerto Rican subjects perceive their important support needs as generally well met by informal support systems composed of friends and families. The subjects are very involved in reciprocal support relationships and attach importance to the satisfaction they get from helping others.

449   Ecklein, J. (1982). Women in the German Democratic Republic:
       impact of culture and social policy. In Giele, J. (Ed.), Women in the
       middle years: current knowledge and directions for research and
       policy, pp. 151-197. New York: John Wiley & Sons, 283p.

This chapter examines the effects of social policies in socialist Germany "on women's education, occupation, leadership, and family life." Most significant freedoms found are the right to employment, advancement, and further education, the right to determine the number and spacing of their children, and the right to marry, divorce or remain single with or without children with no alteration in social status. "Women are no longer dependent on men for either social status or economic support."

450   Fleishman, R., & Shmueli, A.   (1984).   Patterns of informal social
       support of the elderly: an international comparison. Gerontologist,
       24(3), 303-312.

The elderly of Baka, a Jerusalem neighborhood, receive storing, family-oriented informal
support and minimal participation in support activities by non-relatives.

451   Gibson, M.   (1985-1986).   Older women: an overlooked resource in
       development. Ageing International, 12(4), 12-15+.

Both developed and developing countries are asked to incorporate and expand ways to use
the major increase of people 80 and over, "most of whom are and will continue to be
women."

452   Goldstein, M., Schuler, S., & Ross, J.   (1983).   Social and economic
       forces affecting intergenerational relations in extended families in a
       third world country: a cautionary tale from South Asia. Journal of
       Gerontology, 38(6), 716-724.

Male and female high-caste Hindu adults 59 to 95 in Kathmandu, Nepal, are interviewed
regarding social relations within their families.

453   Koyano, W., Shibata, H., Nakazato, K., Haga, H., Suyama, Y., &
       Matsuzaki, T.   (1988).   Prevalence of disability in instrumental activities
       of daily living among elderly Japanese. Journal of Gerontology, 43(2),
       41-45.

The prevalence of disability in instrumental activities of daily living among elderly
residents in an urban Japanese community is studied.   Generally, there was low prevalence
of disability was low, but increased significantly with age.   Controlling for age, the
prevalence was higher in females than in males, except in preparing meals.

454   Lalive d'Espinay, C. J.   (1985).   Depressed elderly women in
       Switzerland: an example of testing and of generating theories.
       Gerontologist, 16(6), 597-604.

In this Swiss study, a high proportion of farm women are depressed because of culture
shock between traditional values and the realities of everyday life.   Life histories are used
to supplement the survey data.

455   Lesnoff-Caravaglia, G.   (1982).   The Black "granny" and the Soviet
       "babushka":   commonalities and contrasts. In Manuel, R. C.   (Ed.),
       Minority aging: sociological and psychological issues, pp. 109-114.
       Westport, Connecticut: Greenwood Press.

Both "granny" and "babushka" have "evolved as pivotal roles" for older women "to provide
balance for the survival cycle of generations."   These roles have developed from an
economic basis and with activity centered on the rearing of grandchildren.

456   **Lewis, M.   (1982).   Aging in the People's Republic of China. International Journal of Aging and Human Development, 15(2), 79-105.**

Since the Communist government rule in 1949, there has been a steady increase of women in the labor force. All women under 40 have been required to work since 1958. Very few older women have any leadership roles or policymaking power above the local level.

457   Mazess, R., & Forman, S.   (1979).   Longevity and age exaggeration in Vilcabamba, Ecuador. Journal of Gerontology, 34(1), 94-98.

Women are included in the study of an Ecuadorian population noted for extreme ages (over 100 years). There was no evidence of increased longevity in the Vilcabamba population.

458   Norman, D., Murphy, J., Gilligan, C., & Vasdudev, J.   (1981-1982). Sex differences and interpersonal relationships: a cross-sectional sample in the U.S. and India.   International Journal of Aging and Human Development, 14(4), 291-306.

Sixty-two subjects, 19 to 75, from the United States and India, are studied as to kinds of relationships which they identify as important. Females identify more relationships than males. At age 35, both sexes converge on the number of relationships mentioned. Age also is the low point in the number of relationships mentioned by both sexes, while subjects aged 50 to 75 represent the high point in number of relationships. American subjects say parents and immediate family represent their relationships more often, while Indian subjects respond extended and collateral kin more often as important relationships.

459   Pampel, F., & Park, S.   (1986).   Cross-national patterns and determinants of female retirement.   American Journal of Sociology, 91(4), 932-955.

Hypotheses relating to effects of industrial development, social security growth, sex stratification, and family structure and fertility on cross-national patterns of female retirement are tested.

460   Togonu-Bickersteth, F.   (1986).   Age identification among Yoruba aged. Journal of Gerontology, 41(1), 110-113.

The study of the influence of chronological age, number of grandchildren, and life satisfaction on age identification of Yoruba residents 55 and older in Ile-Ife (in western Nigeria) shows a strong positive correlation between chronological age and age identification for both men and women.

461   Tracy, M.   (1987).   Credit-splitting and private pension awards in divorce: a case study of British Columbia, Canada.   Research on Aging, I(1), 148-159.

Examines the experience of earnings-splitting under the Canada Pension Plan and private pension assignments in British Columbia. Author concludes that "a positive impact on the level of retirement income of divorced women will probably only result from a mandatory, not voluntary, system," that "a comparably low incidence of future private pension awards to women as part of the property settlement is related to prevailing judicial attitudes, length of marriage, and the preference of women for immediate payment of cash or in-kind benefits.

Films

462   Post, L., & Rosow, E. (1983). Doctora. Natazumi Productions.

Illustrates life and social conditions in Bolivia through the story of a German woman, who went to La Paz, Bolivia, in 1940.

Dissertations

463   Choi, S-J. (1984). Modernization and social integration of the aged into the family in Korea. Unpublished doctoral dissertation, Case Western Reserve University, 1980.

The effect of factors salient to modernization on the social integration of the aged into their families in contemporary Korean society is studied. Sex difference did not have a direct influence upon social integration, but had indirect influence through interaction with other factors.

464   Kadom, W. (1984). A comparison of influences that motivate a desire in women participants age 15-45 from rural and urban areas of Iraq to continue their education after completing People's School. Unpublished doctoral dissertation, Kansas State University, 212p.

Two hundred female students in rural and urban areas of Baghdad, Iraq, compose the sample. The majority continuing their education were from urban areas and with high grade point averages.

465   Koo, J. (1982). Korean women in widowhood. Unpublished doctoral dissertation, University of Missouri-Columbia, 269p.

The consequences of modernization on the social integration of widows in a modernizing society, Korea, shows older urban widows are less integrated, depend on their children, and have no authority over their family members. Mainly socioeconomic factors lead to the lower integration of urban widows. Older rural widows have higher degrees of social integration.

466   Rosenberger, N. (1984). Middle-aged Japanese women and the meanings of the menopausal tradition. Unpublished doctoral dissertation, University of Michigan, 437p.

The changing meanings of female aging in Japan are interpreted through the ideas used to explain menopausal distress. The middle-aged women who overcome their menopausal problems through hobbies, part-time work, and friendships, represent a new view of the adult self who finds her "worth" in individual-centered activities outside of the household.

467   Sternberg, M.   (1982).   **The long-term adaptations of young and middle-aged widows to the loss of a spouse.**   Unpublished doctoral dissertation, Columbia University Teachers College, 153p.

Sixteen widows with dependent children in the United States and Israel are interviewed, with regard to changes and adjustment as a result of the losing of a spouse. Problems from the loss last well beyond the initial crisis.

Middle Age

Books

468   Berglas, C.   (1983).   <u>Mid-life crisis.</u>   Lancaster, Pennsylvania: Technomic Publishing Company, 109p.

The book covers mid-life crisis, menopause, retirement, living with children, uprooting, widowhood. There is no special focus on women; rather there is a broad look at middle age and old age of both men and women.

469   Brown, J., Kerns, V., & contributors. (1985). <u>In her prime: a new view of middle-aged women.</u> South Hadley, Massachusetts: Bergin & Garvey Publishers, Inc., 217p.

Descriptive data on middle-aged women in diverse cultures--from primitive tribes to late industrial societies--are presented. Anthropological reports on the status of women, their rights and their daily routines during their middle years are provided. Middle-aged women are described in developmental, cross-cultural, and evolutionary perspective. Ranging from concepts of sexuality and social control to motherhood and nurture to a developmental psychological perspective of older women, the articles report on cultures of the !Kung, Bakgaladai, New Guinea, Comoro Islands, Belize, Israel, China, Malaysia, Canada, and the Sudan.

470   Conway, J., & Conway, S. (1983). <u>Women in midlife crisis.</u> Wheaton, Illinois: Tyndale House Publishers, Inc., 394p.

Written from pastoral and counseling background, the book provides pragmatic approaches for women to deal effectively with such mid-life crises as career development/career change, self-esteem, parenting, marital satisfaction. Includes a discussion of preventive techniques.

471   Dale, V. (1984). Women at mid-life: moving beyond stereotypes.
       Liguori, Missouri: Liguori Publications, 79p.

For mid-life women, the book covers developing potential, accepting feelings, becoming
sensitive to oneself and others.

472   Fine, I., (1983). Milidfe and its rite of passage ceremony. San Diego,
       California: Woman's Institute for Continuing Jewish Education, 67p.

The focus is on midlife among Jewish women and promoting creative and productive work
during this period.

473   Golan, N. (1986). The perilous bridge: helping clients through mid-
       life transitions. New York: The Free Press, 255p.

This book considers the emotional, physical, and familial changes occurring for many
individuals during the transition to late middle age, and offers advice on appropriate
treatment of crises which often arise at this period. it begins with an overview of various
perspectives on late midlife, including women's perspective.

474   Hepworth, M., & Featherstone, M. (1982). Surviving middle age.
       Oxford, England: Basil Blackwell Publisher, Limited.

Two sociologists present a sympathetic perspective of middle age, focusing on spiritual and
physical vigor and renewal. The entire book looks at both men and women and attitudes
toward aging. A humorous, but useful, questionnaire on mid-life is included.

475   Kubelka, S. (1982). Over 40 at last. New York: Macmillan, 237p.

This book presents a look at why people are afraid of age and aging, and concludes that
"the world...belongs to people with maturity, personality, character, and experience."

476   Markey, J. (1984). How to survive your high school reunion...and
       other mid-life crises. Chicago: Contemporary Books, Inc., 157p.

Humorous, philosophical vignettes from the author's experiences dealing with school class
reunions, family relationships, reaching middle age, and aging parents are presented.

477   Pellegrino, V. Y. (1981). The other side of thirty: the new
       breakthrough decade in a woman's life. New York: Rawson, Wade
       Publishers, Inc., 241p.

This report of questionnaires and interviews of over 1,000 American women in their thirties
finds these women discovering new opportunities. Discussion includes motherhood after
thirty, the success syndrome, the joy of money, the lesbian experience, singlehood.

478   Rogers, N. (1980). <u>Emerging woman: a decade of midlife transitions.</u>
      Point Reyes, California: Personal Press, 201p.

The book is a psychological and personalized perspective of a woman's journey, with an
emphasis on communication and honesty. The author shares what she has learned from her
own life experiences and explores her attitudes and experiences with men and with women.

479   Wax, J. (1979). <u>Starting in the middle.</u> New York: Holt, Rinehart
      and Winston, 204p.

Woody Allen's statement, "Life must be understood backward" summarizes this book. A
self-examination by the author and experiences of others in midlife are presented in a
humorous vein.

480   Westoff, L. (1980). <u>Breaking out of the middle-age trap.</u> New York:
      The New American Library, Inc., 347p.

One hundred case histories of women who have faced the challenges of middle age are
provided, with discussion of tensions, physical stresses, growth, work, politics, upward
mobility, business, jobsearch, education, transition planning, breakdowns, and breakups.
"This book is primarily about those women who are facing the challenge, breaking out of
their used up past and doing what they have secretly always wanted to do."

481   Wood, D. (1981). <u>Middle age and other spreads.</u>   Cape Coral,
      Florida: D. Wood, 126p.

A humorous, personal perspective of middle age is given.

Films

482   Greenberg & O'Hearn Productions (Producers). (1979). <u>Four women
      over 40.</u>

This film gives positive role models, emphasizing the importance of physical and mental
activity at all ages.

483   Paulist Productions (Producer). (No date). <u>Last of the great male
      chauvinists.</u> (Also available in videocassette).

Ann faces the "empty nest" period of middle age, with her children gone and with no
interests outside her home.

484   <u>Transitions: caught at midlife.</u> (1980). (Video).

This story of marriage describes a trapped wife, a May/December affair, and a stale
marriage.

Documents

485   United States Congress, Select Committee on Aging, U.S. House of
Representatives. (1980). The status of mid-life women and options for
their future, 34p.

This publication reports a comprehensive study, by the Subcommittee on Retirement
Income and Employment, of national policies affecting midlife women. The report
concludes that "economic independence and security for older women are attainable, if
educational and vocational opportunities are accessible, especially in the middle years."

486   United States House of Representatives, Select Committee on Aging and
Subcommittee on Retirement Income and Employment.   (1978).
Women in midlife--security and fulfillment, 333p.

This annotated bibliography includes books, journal articles, and government publications
on women in midlife. The majority of the citations are from the 1970s. Subjects covered
include social roles, work, education, pensions, discrimination, housing, mental health, and
political participation.

Dissertations

487   Moore, E. (1982). Apparel purchasing problems of the middle-aged
woman. Unpublished doctoral dissertation, Texas Woman's University,
104p.

Two hundred and twenty-two females, aged 35 to 60, comprise the sample. Variation in
problems with quality [of apparel] due to difficulty purchasing jackets, stores where clothes
were purchased, and weight loss after age 35 are described. Contributing to known
variation in problems with price were figure type/size, white ethnic group, and price paid
for a dress.

488   Rabin, L. (1983). An investigation of early adult and midlife adult life
structure for women living a neotraditional life pattern. Unpublished
doctoral dissertation, University of Pittsburgh, 213p.

The study describes adult years for women who follow a "neotraditional" life pattern--
working followed by full-time homemaking and, then, working while homemaking. In the
midlife phase, women modified their competency needs, experienced a need for self-
expression, expanded their self-assertion and self-esteem, maintained a social network, and
considered great life issues.

General

Books

489   Bell, M. (Ed.) (1986). <u>Women as elders: images, visions, and issues.</u>
New York: Harrington Park Press, also Haworth Press, 90p.

A collection of chapters about issues affecting older women. Topics include "crones,"
older black women, aging religious sisters, retirement planning and women business
owners, health care, and policy.

490   Block, M., Davidson, J., & Grambs, J. D. (1981). <u>Women over forty:</u>
<u>visions and realities.</u> New York: Springer Publishing Company, 157p.

Research about older women. Identifies gaps in the research literature on the middle-aged
and older woman.

491   Borenstein, A. (1983). <u>Chimes of change and hours: views of older</u>
<u>women in 20th-century America.</u> Rutherford: Fairleigh Dickinson
University Press, 518p.

Older women as seen through social science and literature and through oral histories and
memoirs. Extensive historical survey of the roles of older women throughout history and
in various cultures.

492   Borenstein, A. (1982). <u>Older women in 20th-century America.</u> New York:
Garland Publishers, 351p.

Topics include activism against ageism, social criticism, autobiographies, creativity and
productivity in later life, arts and the elderly, cross-cultural perspectives, gerontology,
housing and living environments, life-span development, literature, middle age, novels and
novellas by and about older women, oral histories, personal documents of older women,
psychological perspectives on aging, short stories by and about older women, social and
economic issues, sociological perspectives, selected bibliographies.

493   Boyle, S. (1983). The desert blooms: a personal adventure in growing old creatively. Nashville: Abington Press, 207p.

An account of the author's personal experience with aging written to help older readers understand their own experiences and improve their self-images.

494   Cohen, L. (1984). Small expectations: society's betrayal of older women. Toronto: McClelland and Stewart Limited, 228p.

Analyzes the causes and prejudices against women as they age, criticizing "society's denial of women's needs and of its failure to preserve basic human rights." Includes stories of older women who have battled society against becoming second-class citizens. Author surveys existing political remedies and calls for destruction of the social prejudices toward aging individuals.

495   Datan, N., & Lohmann, N. (Eds.) (1980). Transitions of aging. New York: Academic Press, 221p.

Proceedings of the First West Virginia University gerontology Conference, which focused on rural aged and aging women. Contributors cover adult cognition, life satisfaction, physical activity and health, competence, intergenerational relations, widowhood, clinical psychology of later life, economic status, and institutionalization.

496   Dolan, E., & Gropp, D. (1984). The mature woman in America: a selected annotated bibliography, 1979-1982. Washington, D.C.: The National Council on the Aging, Inc., 122p.

Over 420 items on mature women in America and the policies which affect them. Materials "stress statistics and research, both of which reflect current greatly increased interest in women and their roles in modern America."

497   Edelstein, B., & Segedin, L. (1977). Age is becoming: an annotated bibliography on women and aging. Berkeley: Interface Bibliographers.

A selective bibliography of current literature about the impact of aging on women in contemporary America. General and scholarly publications covering the period 1970-1977 are evaluated from a feminist viewpoint.

498   Fuller, M., & Martin, C. (1980). The older woman: lavender rose or Gray Panther. Springfield, Illinois: Charles C Thomas, Publisher, 343p.

Interdisciplinary and sociological anthology on the problems and needs of older women today. Emphasizes individuality of older women and the continuing (evolving) socialization of women.

499   Hemmings, S. (1985). A wealth of experience: the lives of older women. London: Pandora Press, 181p.

A collection of "personal histories and political commitments," intended "to identify some common roots and shared causes" among women 40 to 65. The book has, according to the author, "a conscious political purpose."

500   Hirschfield, I., & Lambert, T.   (1978).   Audio-visual aids: uses and resources in gerontology. Los Angeles, California: The Ethel Percy Andrus Gerontology Center, 179p.

Evaluations of films, filmstrips, videotapes, slides and audiocassettes on aging.

501   Hollenshead, C., with Ingersoll, B. & Katz, C.   (1977).   Past sixty: the older woman in print and film. Ann Arbor: Institute of Gerontology, University of Michigan, 55p.

Annotated list of 289 selected books, journal and magazine articles, pamphlets and films which focus on women over 60. Topics include widowhood, sexuality, ethnic background, and health.

502   Jacobs, R. (1979). Life after youth. Boston: Beacon Press, 168p.

Presented are discussions of the author's typology of older women--1) nurturers, 2) unutilized nurturers, 3) re-engaged nurturers, 4) chum networkers and leisurists, 5) careerists--employed and unemployed, 6) seekers, 7) faded beauties, 8) doctorers, 9) escapists and isolates, and 10) advocates and assertive older women.

503   Klein, L. (1983). Old, older, oldest. New York: Hastings House, 45p.

A children's book about aging--features a grandmother coming to visit the grandchildren.

504   Lesnoff-Caravaglia, G. (1984). The world of the older woman. New York: Human Sciences Press, Inc., 189p.

Topics include the double stigmata of being female and old, psychosocial problems of older women, social class, abuse, legal issues, institutionalization, widowhood, feminism, older Soviet women, policy directions, and program design.   Multidisciplinary perspective. Assertion of the common interests, problems, and concerns of older women.

505   Maddox, G. (Ed.). (1987). The encyclopedia of aging. New York: Springer Publishing Company, 890p.

Reference work providing succinct explanations for hundreds of concepts related to the aging process and services provided for the elderly. Approximately 500 entries and an extensive bibliography.

506   Markson, E.   (Ed.)   (1983).   Older women.   Lexington, Massachusetts: Lexington Books/D. C. Heath and Company, 351p.

Primary focus of these contributions is on women 60 and older, but the book also includes discussion of changes occurring at 40 and over. "These mid-life events influence and often shape the future course of the remainder of life, although they are by no means all determining."

507   McIlvaine, B., & Mundkur, M., et al.   (1978).   Aging: a guide to reference sources, journals, and government publications.   Storrs, Connecticut: University of Connecticut Library.

General guide to aging-related publications, with section on women.

508   Melamed, E.   (1983).   Mirror, mirror: the terror of not being young. New York: Linden Press/Simon & Schuster, 220p.

Addresses the belief in American society that it is acceptable for men, but not for women, to age. Chapters on fear of aging, neutering, older women and the media, body image, and authenticity.

509   Michigan, University of.   (1975).   No longer young: the older woman in America.   Ann Arbor, Michigan: Institute of Gerontology, University of Michigan, 120p.

Proceedings of the twenty-sixth annual conference on aging--sections on status and stereotypes of older women, mechanisms for change, status of women in the future.

510   Michigan, University of.   (1974).   No longer young: work group reports from the 26th annual conference on aging.   Ann Arbor, Michigan: Institute of Gerontology, University of Michigan, 85p.

Work group summaries from a three-day conference on "Women: life span challenges" at the University of Michigan in 1973.   Covers class and ethnic variations, service needs, volunteerism, media, self-image.

511   Miller, L.   (1979).   Late bloom: new lives for women.   New York: Paddington Press, Ltd., 256p.

Collection of personal stories of women who, in middle age, made a decision to live for themselves based on their individual abilities and interests.   Sections on survivors with style, motherhood, bravery, women supporting women.

512   National Coalition on Older Women's Issues.   (1986).   Midlife and older women: a resource directory.   Washington, D.C.:   National Coalition on Older Women's Issues, 88p.

This directory was developed by the National Coalition on Older Women's Issues as a reference to organizations which provide services or other resources for/on midlife and

older women.   Information is provided on each of the organizations, and organiations are
also classified by topic, such as health care, job development, and income.

513   Painter, C., text; Valois, P., photographs.   (1985).   Gifts of age:
      portraits and essays of 32 remarkable women.   San Francisco,
      California: Chronicle Books, 147p.

Women such as older women's advocate Tish Sommers, photographer Eleanor Lawrence,
flower arrangement designer Haruko Obata, and medicine woman Martha St. John, share
their later years.

514   Peterson, N. (1981).   Our lives for ourselves: women who have never
      married.   New York: G. P. Putnam's Sons, 264p.

Personal stories of women of all ages who have never married--"women who lead lives of
positive autonomy."   Discussion of the quality of their lives, the choices they had to make,
their contentment and their difficulties in a life that is "different."

515   Porcino, J.   (1983)   Growing older, getting better: a handbook for
      women in the second half of life.   Reading, Massachusetts: Addison-
      Wesley Publishing Company, 364p.

Written by the director of The National Action Forum for Midlife and Older Women, this
book combines personal stories, examples, and facts to illustrate the challenges and
opportunities faced by women over 40.   It is divided into information related to family and
personal transitions and to physical changes.   Includes discussion of family roles,
widowhood, finances, health, sexuality, health afflictions, and addictions.

516   Rich-McCoy, L. (1980).   Late bloomer: profiles of women who found
      their true calling.   New York: Harper & Row, 225p.

Stories of mature women who "try something totally different, develop a new life and style
within a responsible carer.   The later bloomer becomes a self-created success."   "How she
did it" listing at the end of each vignette.

517   Rossi, A.   (Ed.).   (1985).   Gender and the life course.   New York:
      Aldine Publishing Company, 368p.

The theme is gender differentiation in a life span framework.   Interdisciplinary collection of
essays on men and women as they are affected by history, culture, demography, economic
and political stratification, and biopsychological changes.   The papers were first presented
in 1983 to the American Sociological Association.   Gender and age are viewed as
maturational factors.

518   Sahara, P. (1977). Media: resources for gerontology. Ann Arbor:
       Institute of Gerontology, University of Michigan, 144p.

Annotated listing of films, filmstrips, videotapes, slides, and audiotapes on aging and
related issues.

519   Seskin, J. (1985). Alone--not lonely: independent living for women
       over fifty. Washington, D.C.: American Association of Retired
       Persons; Glenview, Illinois: Scott, Foresman, Lifelong Learning
       Division, 229p.

Discussion of loneliness, emotional well-being, health needs, social life, holidays, finances,
work, education, housing, leisure time, sexuality. "we are all basically alone. How much
we connect to others is up to us."

520   Seskin, J. (1980). More than mere survival: conversations with
       women over 65. New York: Newsweek Books, 269p.

Stories of 22 women, aged 66 and 97, reveal their lives, their disappointments, and
happinesses. "Each has preserved her zest for living, her self-confidence, and her sense of
humor. Each continues to live actively and productively."

521   Simmons, P. (1976). The president and her sweet old ladies. Boston:
       Branden Press, 81p.

Photographs and narrative on the older women who are part of the "Burton Senior
Citizens"--"the story of all women in this country who are caught in the doubly damning
web of old age and poverty."

522   Sommers, T. (1976). Aging in America: implications for women.
       Washington, D.C.: The National Council on the Aging, Inc., 17p.

Based on the National Council on the Aging Louis Harris and Associates public opinion
study, "The Myth and Reality of Aging in America," the focus is on gender as a variable in
the study. Includes potential effects for public policy and for involvement and action.

523   Stoddard, K. (1983). Saints and shrews: women and aging in
       American popular film. Westport, Connecticut: Greenwood Press,
       174p.

Interpretation of older women in popular film. Evaluates society's attitudes toward aging,
using film to show how some attitudes "are articulated and altered within an artistic
model."

524   Wasserman, P., Koehler, B., & Lev, Y. (Eds.). (1987). Encyclopedia of
       senior citizens information sources. Detroit, Michigan: Gale Research
       Company, 503p.

A bibliographic guide to 13,500 citations for publications, organizations, and other sources of information on about 300 topics related to senior citizens. Includes women as a subject area.

525   Wheelwright, J. (1984). For women growing older. Houston: C. G. Jung Educational Center of Houston, 59p.

The author attempts to show that "a meaningful later life is a by-product of the knowledge, but more importantly, of the conscious or unconscious experience of the animus," the soul or the unconscious.

526   Women Studies Abstracts. (1972). Rush, New York: Rush Publishing Company.

An index to scholarly research on women. Relevant subject headings include: aging, older adults, seniors, middle age, old age survivors insurance, senior women.

527   Words on Aging. (1970). Westport, Connecticut: Greenwood Publishers; Washington, D.C.: U.S. Department of Health, Education, and Welfare, Administration on Aging, 190p.

Glossary of age-related terms.

Articles

528   Costello, M., & Meacham, J. (1980-1981). Sex differences in perception of aging. International Journal of Aging and Human Development, 12(4), 283-290.

Thirty people over 65 were asked to rate the difficulty of 16 events for themselves, other women, and other men. Subjects found difficulty for oneself not as great as they perceived it to be for others.

529   Davis, R. (1987). Images of aging in the media. In Maddox, G. (Ed.), The encyclopedia of aging, pp. 343-344. New York: Springer Publishing Company, 890p.

Discusses images of men versus images of women. Women are seen far less often, in the media, than are men, as both age. When women are portrayed, it's more apt to be a negative portrayal. Beyond middle age, women are seen in the nurturing role more often than any other role.

530   Holahan, C. (1981). **Lifetime achievement patterns, retirement and life satisfaction of gifted aged women.** Journal of Gerontology, 36(6), 741-749.

Relationship of lifetime achievement patterns and retirement to life satisfaction for 352 gifted aging women from Terman's study of the gifted.

531   Liang, J. (1982). **Sex differences in life satisfaction among the elderly.** Journal of Gerontology, 37(1), 100-108.

A causal model of life satisfaction was proposed and evaluated using four data sets, with a comparison of male and female sub-samples. No systematic sex differences were found in terms of structural parameters; i.e., the same causal mechanism operated among the males and the females.

532   Puglisi, J., & Jackson, D. (1980-1981)   **Sex role identity and self esteem in adulthood.** International Journal of Aging and Human Development, 12(2), 129-138.

Sex role identity and self-esteem were investigated in a sample of 2,069 Ohio State University students, alumni, and employees 17 to 89 years of age. Among both males and females, "psychologically androgynous individuals displayed the highest levels of self-esteem."

533   Sands, J. (1981-1982). **The relationship of stressful life events to intellectual functioning in women over 65.** International Journal of Aging and Human Development, 14(1), 11-22.

Study of 112 women aged 65 to 92. "Stress was found to be related to the ratio used to estimate decline.

534   Steitz, J. (1981-1982). **The female life course: life situations and perception of control.** International Journal of Aging and Human Development, 14(3), 195-204.

Adult male and female subjects perceived the greatest direct personal control or indirect control through the ability to influence powerful others (than did adolescent or retired subjects). Adult females perceived a greater degree of influence on powerful others than did adolescent or retired females, but the same as males of any age status period.

535   Tate, L. (1982). **Life satisfaction and death anxiety in aged women.** International Journal of Aging and Human Development, 15(4), 299-306.

Life satisfaction was predicted by number of friends, good health, and by having fewer offspring living in the same city. Health problems, change in living conditions, and relatively high educational level were predictors of death anxiety.

536   Turner, B.   (1987).   Psychotherapy: age and sex stereotypes.   In
      Maddox, G. (Ed.), The encyclopedia of aging, pp. 551-552.   New York:
      Springer Publishing Company, 890p.

Gender   differences   not   explcitly   addressed   by   many   geropsychologists   and
geropsychiatrists.   Reports a 1982 study which suggests that "sexism is a major component
in the neglect of the elderly by mental health professionals."

537   Turner, B.   (1987).   Self-concepts: sex differences.   In Maddox, G.
      (Ed.), The encyclopedia of aging, pp. 591-592.   New York: Springer
      Publishing Company, 890p.

The literature reveals that, in all age cohorts, American women tend to have lower self-
esteem than do men.   In late middle age, women benefit in enhanced self-esteem from
"apparent shifts toward a more 'masculine' and less 'feminine' self-concept."   As they
move from middle age to old age, both women and men are more likely to incorporate
cross-sex characteristics into their self-concepts.

538   Ward, R., Sherman, S., & LaGory, M.   (1984).   Informal networks and
      knowledge of services for older persons.   Journal of Gerontology, 39(2),
      216-223.

Informal networks may provide referral to formal services and may reduce awareness of
formal services by substituting for them.

539   Winogrond, I.   (1981).   A comparison of interpersonal distancing
      behavior in young and elderly adults.   International Journal of Aging
      and Human Development, 13(1), 53-60.

Relationship between sensory deficits in the elderly and their use of personal space in peer
interactions studied.   In comparison of young, white, female college students and elderly,
white females, there were no significant differences in arousal level.

Films

540   Abrahms, H. (Producer).   (No date).   Dear Mr. and Mrs. Bertholf.

Eighty-year-old and 85-year-old husband and wife share their extensive travel experiences
with their children.

541   ACI Films.   (1972).   The art of age.

Profiles four senior citizens, including a 76-year-old sculptress and a woman writer dying
of bone disease.   The emphasis is on activity and positive thoughts of new beginnings.

542 AESOP. (1977). Tillie's philodendron.

Animated allegory about a lonely woman. Represents human need for caring and approval and the effects of anger and hostility.

543 Aging In Our Time Series. (1979). Old is.....

Four men and women who are vigorously active in their seventies, eighties, and nineties illustrate the challenges, frustrations, pleasures, and satisfactions of aging.

544 AIMS. (1978). Crime; senior alert.

Vignettes on ways senior citizens can avoid becoming crime victims. Includes example of preventing a purse snatcher from taking anything of value.

545 Australian Information Service. (1975). Hattie.

Hattie, completely alone at 76, had been very active. Now living in a suburb, she does housework, visits others when she can, "says she doesn't care if she dies tomorrow."

546 Bullfrog Films. (1977). Living the good life with Helen and Scott Nearing.

Helen and Scott, 74 and 93, pianist and economist, quit city life 45 years ago for Vermont, where they have been self-sufficient, involved, balanced, and healthy.

547 Burst-Terranella, F. (1980). Lila. (Also video).

Lila Bonner-Miller, 80, is a practicing psychiatrist, artist, and church leader. She illustrates how one older person continues an active, productive schedule.

548 California, University of. (1983). Dance mask: the world of Margaret Severn. University of California Extension Media Center.

In the early twentieth century, ballerina Margaret Severn tells how she developed choreoraphy for the vaudeville stage, including her trademark mask dance.

549 Chenzira, A. (produced 1975, released 1979). Syvilla: they dance to her dream.

Still montages and interviews with Syvilla Fort, a pioneer black choreographer-teacher. Depicts attempts to give to the next generation certain modern dance traditions despite her "lack of funds, lack of recognition, and the debilitating effects of age and disease."

550 Contemporary Films/McGraw-Hill. (1965). The string bean.

The story of a gaunt older woman and her nurturing of her bean plant.   Illustrates how loneliness may be eased and how defeat may become success.

551   Coolidge, M. (Producer).   (1974).   Old-fashioned woman.

Martha Coolidge's portrait of her grandmother, 87-year-old Mabel Tilton Coolidge.   Self-sufficient and involved in life, Mabel Coolidge reminisces about childhood and gives her views on contemporary issues.

552   Danska, H. (Producer).   (1976).   Miss Larsen: rebel at 90.

A 90-year-old woman traces her life of revolt and self-determination, through hospital and nursing home situations with tranquilizers, restraints, etc.

553   Dean, J. (Producer).   (1980).   The women of Hodson.   (Also video).

Stories of women septuagenarians in the South Bronx who develop and perform original works based on their own life experiences.

554   Edwards, C. (1985).   Song of wool: Vena Tipton's hooked rugs.

Artist Vena Tipton, 91, weaves stories of her life into her rug and tapestry creations.

**555   Film Dallas I and Bountiful Film Productions   (Producers).   (1986).
          The trip to Bountiful.**

An elderly woman who lives with her son and daughter-in-law in a cramped Houston apartment wants to return to her home in Bountiful, a small country town.   Film depicts her attempts to journey home and to be reconciled with her past.

556   Geltman, S. (1984).   Breaking 100.   Centre Productions.

Illustrates the lives of several centenarian Americans, including Olga Ulke, a Viennese socialite and actress, and Mary Duckworth, once a slave.

557   Giummo, J. (Producer).   (1978).   Shopping bag ladies.

Documentary of shopping bag ladies in New York City.   They are hungry, cold, and isolated, but exhibit fierce independence, a desire to be free, and a goal of living without depending on official charity.

558   Golan, M. & Globus, Y. (1985).   Grace Quigley.

Grace Quigley is a poor, but strong-willed, woman who sets up a business to provide death with dignity for the older person.

559   Gordon-Kerchoff Productions, Inc. (Producer). (1980). What do you see, nurse?

Reconstructs the life of an elderly woman patient in a nursing home. Based on a poem by Phyllis McCormack, a nurse in Scotland.

560   Granada TV International (Producer). (No date). Death by request.

Meg Murphy, 78, argues her right to end a life no longer meaningful to her.: concerned that multiple sclerosis may disable her so she can't end her life when she wants to, her goal is to repeal the English law which makes assisting someone to end his/her own life a criminal act.

561   Greenberg & O'Hearn Productions (Producer). (1979). Four women over 80.

Four older women show successful responses to aging through physical activity, continuing education, social involvement, and gainful employment.

562   Grandma's bottle village. (1982).

Grandma Tressa Prisbrey, 84, built her first bottle house to hold 17,000 pencils. The interiors of her 15 houses are documented and displayed as vivid examples of 20th-century folk art.

563   Guidance Films (Producer) (1976). The transformation of Mabel Wells. (Also available in videocassette).

Cranky, complaining Mabel Wells returns home from a six-week hospitalization to find cards, gifts, etc., from people she thought had never even noticed her. her reaction to people's response to her illness are seen.

564   Hammer, B. (1979). Dream age.

Seventy-year-old lesbian feminist sends out her forty-year-old self on a quest and meets aspects of her personality.

565   Highlight Productions, Ltd. (Producer). (1974). Granny's quilts.

Mrs. Catherine Scott shows how she makes patchwork quilts. Examples of her work when young and in her advanced age are shown.

566   Hill, J., Anderson, E., & Museum of the City of New York. (Producer). (1950). Grandma Moses.

A documentary on Grandma Moses, a self-taught artist who began painting in her seventies.

567   Holt, N. (Producer). (1974). Underscan. (Also video).

Film is based on letters about the passage of time received by the artist from her Aunt Ethel. Nancy Holt reads "her aunt's descent into old age."

568   Hubley, F., & Hubley Studios (Producers). (Produced 1975, released 1980). Everybody rides the carousel--"the later years."

Animation with two contrasting elderly couples--one very enthusiastic, one complaining.

569   Hungaro-film (Producer). (1973). The old woman.

Humorous animation about an older woman who is too busy living to go with Death when he arrives. Death finally collapses in humiliation and the woman covers the corpse.

570   Kaw Valley Films. (1980). Daisy Cook remembers.

Daisy Cook describes farm life in the American Midwest through her "modern primitive" paintings.

571   Keneholistic Foundation (Producer). (Produced 1979, released 1980). Living time--Sarah Jesup talks on dying.

Sarah Jesup, 41, in her last three months of life, discusses death as a reality--defines her priorities, discusses living wills, and explains death to her children.

572   Lady in motion: a portrait of Miss Agnes Hammond and friends. (1982).

Profile of a 72-year-old independent woman rancher and artist living in the foothills of the Canadian Rockies.

573   Long, J., & National Film Board of Canada. (produced 1979, released 1980). Poison ivy. (Also video).

Description of the very active life of Ivy Granstrom, who lost most of her vision through insufficient care at birth. She discusses her career as a nurse's aide before she retired.

574   Michigan, University of. (1978). The older woman: issues.

Slide-tape program to trigger discussion on attitudes about aging and older women, widowhood, retirement, etc. Includes a synchronized audio-cassette and a user's manual.

575   Miller, F. (Producer). (1979). Portraits of aging.

Presents a positive view of aging. Shows men and women "from all walks of life, active, vibrant and with zest for living."

576   Mokin, A., Productions (Producer). (1976). Ruth Stout's garden.
       (Also available videocassette).

Ruth Stout, in her tenth decade, "no dig/no work" gardener, writer, shares her memories.
She is still an active gardener, enjoying gardening in the nude in her earlier years. At 16,
she smashed saloons with Carrie Nation in the drinking prohibition crusade.

577   Mouris, C., & Leverington, S. (1977). The detour.

Catherine Hamilton, 83, dying in a hospital, wants peace and dignity, and resents the staff's
efforts to keep her alive.

578   National Film Board of Canada (Producer). (1970). The past--the
       present--the future.

Olga Spence, a 63-year-old widow and retired postmistress, discusses the life she has led in
Newfoundland.

579   National Film Board of Canada. (1983). Portrait of an artist as an old
       lady.

Feminist perspective on painter Paraskeva Clark, 80, "outspoken and funny."

580   National Film Board of Canada and Contemporary Films/McGraw-Hill
       (Producers). (1966). Where Mrs. Whalley lives.

Mrs. Whalley, young-looking, attractive, physically healthy, but with mental deterioration, is
treated by others as a pest. She retreats to her past.

581   O'Connell, P., & the Pennsylvania State University Television
       (Producers). (1975). The final, proud days of Elsie Wurster.

Depicts the last 44 days of Elsie Wurster's life. She is shown as undespairing and full of
dignity. Her interactions with visitors and staff and in therapy are seen. She shares her
feelings and fears and memories.

582   Opequon Productions (Producer). (No date). Off my rocker. (Video).

Clara Cassidy, 78, a West Virginia newspaper columnist, shares her positive, upbeat
approach to growing old.

583   Ore, D., & KUTV Dist. Films, Inc. (Producers). (1976). The history
       of Miss Annie Anderson. (Also available in videocassette).

Ninety-four-year-old Annie Anderson has used memories, her father's journal, old
photographs and letters, to write her history--from arriving in Utah in a covered wagon to
homesteading, etc.

584   Phoenix Films (1973). **Peege.**

Peege, a blind, stroke-crippled grandmother, is visited in the nursing home by her grandson, who tries to "connect" with her through his memories of happier times they've spent together.

585   Phoenix Films. (1980). **Poison ivy.**

Story of Ivy Granstrom, left with very little vision, but who leads a very energetic life--jogging, skiing, gardening, etc.

586   Phoenix Films, Inc. (No date). **Thank you m'am.**

Based on a short story by Langston Hughes about the meaningful meeting between an older black woman and a black youth.

587   Pickering, M. (Producer). (1972). **The Millstone Sewing Center.**

Film tells how a rural community in Letcher County, Kentucky, organized the Millstone Sewing Center under the effective and successful leadership of Mabel Kiser. "The center employs women as seamstresses, gives away clothes to needy families, operates a lunch program, and serves as an information and referral center."

588   Porter, N., & WGBH-TV (Producers). (No date). **Older and bolder.**

The focus is on a small group of older women in Cambridge, Massachusetts, who meet weekly to share joys and problems.   While these women have faced problems and loneliness, they have taken control of their own lives.

589   Prince, N., & Otter Productions (Producers). (Produced 1978, released 1979). **Ruth Page: an American original.** (Also video).

The life of dancer, choreographer, and director Ruth Page from her Midwest childhood through her present teaching and daily practice at the barre are presented.

590   Rhodes, L., & Murphy, M. (Producers). (1978). **They are their own gifts.** (Also video).

Biographies of three American artists--poet Muriel Rukeyser, painter Alice Neel, and choreographer Anna Sokolow.

591   Rocky Mountain Productions (Producer). (1974). **Antonia: a portrait of the woman.**

Antonia Brico, 73, symphony conductor, is profiled.

592   Shadow City Productions.   (1980).   What are they doing to the cat lady?

Documentary on a 60-year-old woman who lives alone in her house with 40 cats.

593   Shands, A., Production, & WAVE-TV   (Producers).   (No date).   All your parts don't wear out at the same time.

Members of "Senior Player" drama group present skits from their lives. "The rewards of their risks can be seen in their own lives and in the faces of their appreciative audiences."

594   She loved the land.   (1977).

Picture of Emma Garrod, 93. This is the oral history of a pioneer-farming community in the Santa Cruz mountains of California.

595   Shirley, R. (Producer).   (1969).   Resonant.
Montage of still photos showing a day in the life of an elderly grandmother.

596   Simon, J.   (1973).   Nana: un portrait.

The filmmaker's grandmother, Nana, age 80, is profiled. Nana looks back at her life from a chair in her New York apartment.

597   Smith, L., & Horwitz, L. (Producers).   (1982).   Where did you get that woman?

Portrait of an aging washroom matron who works in a very nice entertainment district and who lives in the ghetto. Her autobiographical reminiscences show her determination and survival instincts.

598   Stanford University, Department of Communications   (Producer). (1972).   You don't die here.

Impressionistic documentary showing Death Valley as "a cruel and sublime landscape in which a few old people live out their lives." An old woman wanders through the ruins of a mining town and remembers the "glory days" of the town.

599   Tan, H. (Producer).   (1980).   A lady named Baybie.

Documentary on 64-year-old Baybie Hoover, a blind singer who "pitched" her way from Wichita, Kansas, to New York City by singing religious songs with a tin cup in her hand.

600   Taylor, R.   (1981).   For old and young alike.   (Video).

Profile of Boulder, Colorado's poet laureate, Florence Becker Lennon, 86, political activist, author and writer, children's poetry workshop organizer, and humanitarian.

601   Teleculture, Inc. (Producer). (1982). **Alberta Hunter: blues at the cookery.** (Also video).

Profile of an 87-year-old black woman blues singer. A nurse, she gave up music for 20 years and re-started her musical career at 82.

602   Trigger Films on Aging (1971). **To market, to market, Mrs. P., The center, Dinner time, and Tagged.**

Five vignettes about aging: a lady with food stamps at a grocery, an elderly volunteer losing a job, intergenerational conflict, solitary supper, and losing furniture.

603   UMMRC (Producer). (1978). **What we have.**

Portrays the activities of grandparents when they visit an elementary school.

604   Vanden, J. (Producer). (1982). **Take a stand.**

A "role-played documentary," based on the real case of an older woman, victim of a mugging, who testifies in court against her attacker.

605   Washington, University of. (1982). **Exploring aging.** University of Washington Instructional Media Center.

Interview with a 91-year-old woman. Advice provided about dealing with aged people.

606   Wengraf, S., Rudnick, C., Dobkin, D., & Red Hen Films (Producers). (1977). **Love it like a fool.**

At 76, Malvina Reynolds "proves that age has only increased her integrity, insight, and humanism." She performs and manages record and publishing companies "with vigor and excitement."

607   WNED-TV (Producer). (1977). **Age is a woman's issue.** (Video).

Tish Sommers, co-founder of the Displaced Homemakers Network [then co-coordinator of NOW's Task Force on Older Women] discusses: age discrimination's effects on older women, displaced homemakers, and societal attitudes toward the older woman.

608   WNED-TV (Producer). (1977). Age is becoming. (Video).

Advantages of growing older and what to do about the disadvantages are discussed by Lydia Bragger, Gray Panthers; Marjory Collins, Prime Time; and Tish Sommers, Co-coordinator of NOW's Task Force on Older Women.

609   Woo who: May Wilson. (1969).

Presents the story of May Wilson, 63, "wife-mother-housekeeper-cook," as she moves from terrified lack of confidence (after her husband left her) to self-assurance as an artist.

610   Zanuck, R., Brown, D., & Zanuck, L. (1986). Cocoon.

Fantasy on dream of recovered youth by cast of older men and women, illustrating direct and indirect effects of the youthful rejuvenation.

Documents

611   U.S. Bureau of Labor Statistics. (1978). Where to find BLS statistics on women.

Statistical summaries of statistics on women, especially in the field of employment, which are available from the Bureau of Labor Statistics. The document provides information on how to acquire the data.

612   U.S. Congress. House. Select Committee on Aging. (1982). Problems of aging women, 157p.

Covers economic concerns, health care, widowhood, pensions, social activity, health insurance, rural aging, displaced homemakers.

613   U.S. Congress. Senate. Special Committee on Aging, American Association of Retired Persons, Federal Council on Aging, Administration on Aging. (1988). Aging America: trends and projections, 1987-88 edition. Washington, D.C.: U.S. Department of Health and Human Services, 186p.

Includes current statistical data on older women, especially as contrasted with older men, in such areas as economic status, retirement trends and labor force participation, health status and health services utilization, social characteristics, and international perspectives.

614   U.S. Congress. Senate. Special Committee on Aging. (1985). America in transition: an aging society, 1984-85 edition, 98p.

An information paper reporting demographic information on America's aging population with respect to geographic distribution and mobility, economic status, retirement trends and labor force participation, health status and health services utilization, social characteristics, and federal outlays benefiting the elderly.

615   **U.S. Department of Health, Education, and Welfare, National Institute on Aging, and National Institute of Mental Health. (1979). The older woman: continuities and discontinuities, 56p.**

Report of a 1978 workshop designed to stimulate the interest of researchers in questions currently relevant to the lives of older women and to generate a future research agenda for two sponsoring institutes.

616   **U.S. National Commission on the Observance of International Women's Year. (1976). Older women: a workshop guide, 39p.**

Provides guidelines designed to assist in setting up a workshop on older women. Includes a fact sheet on problems of older women, suggested goals for workshops, recommendations for the National Conference on the Observance of International Women's Year and other groups, lists of enclosures, publications, films, and possible speakers and panel members.

Dissertations

617   **Bearon, L. (1982). No great expectations: the nature of life satisfaction in a sample of elderly women. Unpublished doctoral dissertation, Duke University, 148p.**

The objective of this study was to identify factors which older women take into account when making a global assessment of their well-being. Older women, more than middle-aged women, cited health as a source of satisfaction and dissatisfaction, favored maintaining the status quo and preventing deterioration, and spontaneously used social comparisons in evaluating their lives. Middle-aged women more frequently cited personal growth and accomplishments as a meaningful domain of life experience.

618   **Brady, E. (1982). Selected correlates of participants' perceptions of growth in elderhostel programs. Unpublished doctoral dissertation, The University of Connecticut, 178p.**

Examines intellectual and personal-social growth perceived by older students participating in Elderhostel programs. The strongest predictors of perceived growth were level of education, sex, and the Elderhostel college attended.

619   **MacKeracher, D. (1982). A study of the experience of aging from the perspective of older women. Unpublished doctoral dissertation, University of Toronto,.**

The aging experiences of 30 older women were the focus of this study. Inquiry into the explanations which older learners attach to activity, disengagement, continuity, and development theories of aging.

620   Pirnot, K. (1986). Reentry women: a follow-up study of women who enter college at a nontraditional age. Unpublished doctoral dissertation, The University of Owa, 242p.

Longitudinal assessment of 29 reentry women at a private liberal arts college in the midwest. Data on basic life values, academic persistence variables, and thematic needs and press. Findings show a general stability of life values from pre- to post-test conditions.

621   Premo, T. (1983). Women growing old in the New Republic: personal responses to old age, 1785-1835. Unpublished doctoral dissertation, University of Cincinnati, 290p.

Women's personal responses to growing old in the 50 years following American independence. "For women growing old, these years signified growing approbation within the woman's sphere. Although changes in Jacksonian America began to erode the social and religious base of the aging experience, women in the New Republic usually found strong continuity in the prospects and the process of growing old."

622   Teuter, U. (1982). Goal development and activity patterns in a group of elderly women experiencing high life satisfaction. Unpublished doctoral dissertation, University of Pittsburgh, 170p.

Explores connection between high life satisfaction in later years and goal development and related activities in earlier phases for women. "Variables emerging consistently were care for others on an individual [level] and on the collective level, care for self, a stance of positive detachment, openmindedness, effectiveness, and efficiency, the ability to focus on essentials, inner-directedness, a solid centeredness, and a lack of envy and self-righteousness."

Appendix

Primary Libraries Utilized in This Literature Review

Resources of, and staff assistance from, the three library collections listed below were utilized in development of the selected annotated bibliographic references included in this collection.

The Library of Congress
10 First Street, S.E.
Washington, D.C., 20540

The National Council on the Aging Library
600 Maryland Avenue, S.W., West Wing 100
Washington, D.C., 20024

The American Associated of Retired Persons Resource Center
1909 K Street, N.W.
Washington, D.C., 20049

Subject Index

A

Adult children 011
Age discrimination 158, 607
Age identification 460
Age-segregated/
age integrated environments 346
Aging 503
Aging parents 252
Alzheimer's disease 253, 262, 336
Antidiscrimination policies 158, 425, 606
Apparel purchasing 487
Art 521, 565, 566, 572, 579, 590
Asia 378, 399, 402, 452
Asian Americans 378, 399, 402
Attitudes 574
Audio-visual aids 500, 518
Australia 447

B

Babushka 455
Bibliography 496, 497, 501
Blacks 320, 357, 359, 365, 376, 377, 399, 380, 382, 383, 386, 388, 389, 391, 400, 403, 404, 407, 410, 414, 415, 418, 586
Blue-collar jobs 173
Bolivia 462

C

Canada 461
Cardiovascular health 235, 288
Career patterns 175, 187, 190
Caregiving 106, 280
Childlessness 026, 037
Chinese 440, 443, 456
Chronic disease 238, 274
Church-based support 320
Communal housing 330
Coping responses 239
Coping with husband's retirement 191
Crime 544, 604
Cubans 356

D

Death and dying 535, 558, 560, 569, 571, 577, 581, 598
Depression 230, 237, 276, 290, 299, 348, 454
Diabetes 419
Disability 453
Disaster (effects of) 241
Displaced homemakers 178
Divorce 006, 118

E

Economic assistance 125
Economics 121, 138, 144, 147, 148, 150
Economic status of women in the labor market 120
Ecuador 457
Education 464
Elderhostels 618
Encylopedia 505, 524, 527
Ethnicity 350

European Americans 351, 358, 362, 364, 368
European ethnic groups 446
Exercise 294, 299

F

Facelifts　261
Falls 278
Family 038, 042
Farm life 546, 570, 580, 594
Female life course 534
Female veterans 087, 088
Fenwick, Millicent 427
Financial experience 124
Friendships 022, 023, 024, 041, 059, 382

G

Gender differentiation 517
German Democratic Republic 449
German Jewish 385
Gifted women　530
Grandmotherhood 045, 063, 074, 085, 503
Gray Panthers 428, 429
Great-grandmotherhood　066, 071
Greece 104
Guide to references　507

H

Hawaiians　378
Health　215, 219, 220, 221, 225, 226, 228, 229, 233, 234, 241, 242, 246, 247, 248, 256, 263, 271, 272, 285, 291, 293, 295, 584
Health needs 223
Health promotion　218
Health services 267, 268, 378, 403, 404
Hearing impairment 249, 292
Hispanic 051, 349, 354, 363, 369, 372, 373, 390, 396, 406, 415
Home health care　255
Housing 323, 326, 333, 334, 335, 336, 341, 342, 347, 348
Humor 312

I

Images 489, 508, 523, 529
Income maintenance 133, 137, 145
Income (retirement) 126, 127, 129, 139
Independent living 519
India 458
Informal networks　538
Inner city 331
Intergenerational relationships 008, 028, 029, 031, 051, 058, 067, 075, 076, 077, 086, 090, 102, 103, 104, 111, 112, 116, 263, 372, 373, 380, 411, 445, 446, 452, 540
International perspective 437, 439, 441, 442, 450
Interpersonal distance 539
Intimacy　065, 069, 078
Iraq 464
Irish Americans 409
Israel 438, 467
Issues 504
Italian Americans 352, 366, 408

K

Korea 367, 411
Korean Americans 367, 411
Kuhn, Maggie 428, 429

L

Leisure programs　283
Lesbianism 014
Life care facility 327
Life events 002, 032
Life expectancy　370
Life satisfaction 093, 109, 114, 117, 172, 295, 326, 348, 377, 447, 530, 535, 543, 617, 622
Living alone 323, 345, 545
Loneliness 216, 542, 550
Longevity 457

M

Marital separation 030
Marriage 052, 053, 064, 068, 070, 109, 110
Medical care 220, 259
Memory loss 240, 244, 298
Menopause 227, 236, 250, 251, 258, 265, 466
Mental health 086, 222, 224, 246, 254, 266, 277, 358
Mental retardation 287
Middle age 469, 474, 475, 477, 478, 479, 480, 481, 482, 483
Midlife 001, 003, 007, 016, 047, 050, 057, 233

Mid-life careers 153
Mid-life crisis/
mid-life transitions 468,
470, 472, 473, 476, 478,
484, 485, 486, 488
Minority aging 353, 355,
360, 370, 371, 374, 405, 412
Motor performance 245, 284
Music   591, 601, 606

N

Native Americans 361, 387,
391, 392, 395, 397, 398,
416, 419
Nursing home   254, 559
Nutrition 296

O

Occupational segregation 162,
186
Older women 496, 497, 498,
499, 504, 506, 508, 509,
510, 511, 513, 515, 516,
520, 525, 547, 548, 549,
551, 552, 553, 554, 555,
556, 562, 563, 567, 568,
580, 583, 589, 591, 592,
593, 595, 596, 597, 599,
600, 602, 605, 610, 615,
616, 619, 621
Older women/younger men 010,
017, 105
Older women's movement 426
Osteoporosis 257

P

Pacific Asians 402
Pain experience 291
Parenting 039
Pensions   128, 140, 141,
142, 149
Perceptions 493, 528
Pet therapy 243
Physical fitness 279
Physical impairment 281
Policy 430, 431, 432,
433, 434, 435, 436, 522
Poverty 119, 122, 130, 151
Pregnancy 289
Problems 543, 612
Professional women 163,
199, 202, 204, 214
Psychosocial development 097
Public housing 329

Puerto Ricans 417
Puerto Rico 448

R

Race 348
Race differences 242
Rape 264
Re-entry women 091, 152,
154, 161, 181, 182, 620
Religion 312, 315, 316, 317
Religious motivation 318
Religious participation 314
Religious sisters 313, 319, 322
Research 490, 526
Residential relocation 325
Resources 512, 524
Retirement 192, 199, 200,
201, 207, 208, 214, 322, 530
Retirement (attitudes toward)
194, 198, 203, 204
Retirement planning 193, 194,
202, 206, 209, 213
Retirement satisfaction 195,
205, 210, 211, 212
Role conflict 165
Role transition 091, 092, 101
Rural 044, 061, 098, 102,
208, 406

S

Self-concepts 347, 532, 537
Self-esteem 107, 282, 297, 305
Self-identity 056, 073,
079, 095, 099
Senility 260
Senior center utilization 376
Senior Companions 335
Sex differences 197
Sex role identity 532
Sex roles 055, 062
Sexual activity 310
Sexuality 301, 302, 304,
305, 306, 307, 308, 309, 311
Shared housing 346
Shopping-bag women 040, 557
Single-case studies 108
Single room occupancy 332
Single women 027, 089,
334, 514
Social Security 123, 135,
136, 143
Social change 060
Social support 166
Social support patterns 450
Social supports 046, 048, 418

Societal expectations 494
Solar retirement housing 344
Soviet Union 455
Spatial abilities 232
Statistics 611, 613, 614
Stereotypes 471, 536
Strength training 275
Stress 217, 231, 237,
246, 296, 533
Students 091, 097, 100,
103, 189, 412
Successful aging 543, 561,
573, 575, 576, 582, 585, 588, 609
Suicide 242
Swedish 444
Switzerland 454

T

Time persepctive 276
Transitions 495
Type A behavior 286
Typologies 502

U

Unions 176
United States 440, 445,
458, 467

V

Victimization 374

W

White-collar women 203
Widowhood 005, 012, 018,
019, 020, 025, 033, 034,
035, 036,   043, 049, 054,
061, 072, 080, 081, 082,
083, 084, 093, 095, 098,
107, 114, 115, 117, 293,
295, 326, 327, 388, 465,
467, 578
Women business owners 193
Work 155, 156, 157, 159,
160, 164, 166, 168, 169,
170, 171, 172, 179, 183,
184, 185, 188, 375
Work force 180

Y

Yoruba 460

Author Index

A

Abe-Ridder, L. 342
Abrahms, H. 540
Adams, C. 306
Adams, R. 022, 023, 024
Ainlay, S. 314
Alldredge-Marshall, G. 273
Allen, K. 089
Almond, P. 385
Alston, J. 315
Alston, L. 315
Ammer, C. 215
Anderson, D. 027
Anderson, E. 566
Anderson, L. 216
Anderson, R. 090
Antonovsky, A. 438
Arens, D. 025
Artean, D. 406
Ashur, G. 386
Atchley, R. 192
Azibo, M. 152

B

Bachrach, C. 244
Bailey, C. 001
Baldwin, C. 005
Barber, J. 407
Barnett, R. 002
Barnewolt, D. 050
Barr, F. 091
Barresi, C. 035
Baruch, G. 002, 003,
047, 050, 233, 303, 379
Bastida, E. 004, 194,
356, 360
Bearon, L. 617

Becerra, R. 349
Beckman, L. 026
Belgrave, L. 274
Bell, M. 193, 319,
364, 489
Benokraitis, N. 178
Berg, S. 444
Berglas, C. 468
Berit, I. 166
Berkun, C. 229
Berry, J. 230
Birch, E. 323
Birren, J. 217
Black, E. 332
Blazer, D. 316
Block, M. 133, 163,
430, 490
Bloom, A. 249
Boldt, J. 373
Borenstein, A. 491, 492
Boyle, S. 493
Brady, E. 618
Braito, R. 027
Brand, F. 235
Breslau, N. 383
Brodey, J. 153
Brody, E. 028, 029,
086, 164, 264, 445
Brooks-Gunn, J. 003,
047, 050, 233, 303, 379
Brown, B. 092
Brown, D. 610
Brown, J. K. 469
Brown, J. N. 005
Brown, R. 275
Brown, S. 250
Budoff, P. 218
Burdeau, G. 387
Burnford, P. 251
Burnford, Z. 251

Burst-Terranella, F. 547
Busch, S. 245

C

Cahn, A. 431
Campbell, R. 334, 445
Campbell, S. 231
Capozzoli, M. 408
Carnochan, D. 252
Carp, F. 324
Carr, M. 276
Carrell, I. 068
Carrell, O. 068
Cartland, B.
Cassidy, M. 165, 210
Cauhape, E. 006
Chappell, N. 350
Chase, D. 253
Chatters, L. 320, 357
Chenzira, A. 549
Chiriboga, D. 030
Choi, K. 367
Choi, S-J. 463
Christensen, D. 324
Clark, L. 146
Clary, F. 093
Clement, C. 321
Coburn, K. 007
Coe, R. 043
Cohen, D. 232
Cohen, J. H. 374
Cohen, J. L. 355, 361
Cohen, J. Z. 007
Cohen, L. 494
Cohler, B. 008, 358, 446
Cokin, L. 277
Collette, J. 447
Connors, D. 409
Conway, J. 470
Conway, K. 359
Conway, S. 470
Cook, S. 312
Coolidge, M. 551
Costello, M. 528
Costley, D. 051
Coyle, J. 193, 194
Coyne, A. 230
Craven, R. 278
Cruz-Lopez, M. 448
Cutler, S. 424

D

Dale, V. 471
Damrosch, S. 302
Danigelis, N. 326
Danska, H. 552
Datan, N. 438, 495

Davidson, J. 179
Davidson, J. 430, 490
Davis, L. 264
Davis, R. 529
Davison, J. 009
Dawson, D. 244
Dean, J. 553
De Guilio, R. 095
Deimling, G. 328
De Lago, L. 094
DeLorey, C. 233
Demetrakopoulos, S. 365
Depner, C. 166
Derenski, A. 010
Dilworth-Anderson, P. 360
Dissinger, K. 119
Dobkin, D. 606
Dolan, E. 496
Doliva, L. 096
Doress, P. 219
Dorfman, L. 195
Driedger, L. 350

E

Eckels, E. 065
Eckert, J. 325
Ecklein, J. 449
Edelstein, B. 220
Edelstein, B. 497
Edwards, C. 554
Edwards, E. 361
Eggers, J. 279
Egginton, M. 221
Ekerdt, D. 196
Endicott, J. 265
Engle, V. 234
Erdwins, C. 031
Essex, M. 239

F

Fallo-Mitchell, L. 032
Featherstone, M. 474
Feil, E. 254
Feinson, M. 033
Fengler, A. 326
Ferraro, K. 034, 035
Figart, D. 120
Fillenbaum G. 197
Fine, I. 472
Finkelstein, L. 097
Firestone, C. 208
Fitting, M. 280
Fleishman, R. 450
Florence, M. 309
Ford, A. 224, 383
Forman, S. 457
Franks, V. 222

Fredericks, S. 154
Freedman, R. 223
Friedman, R. 191
Friedman, S. 281
Friday, P. 098
Frye, L. 211
Fuchs, E. 300
Fulcomer, M. 028, 029
Fuller, M. 315, 316, 330, 332, 498

G

Gagnier, D. 343
Gelfand, D. 266, 362, 430
Gellert, J. 182
Geltman, S. 556
Gentry, M. 036
George, L. 197
Gibeau, J. 183
Gibson, M. 439, 451
Giele, J. 420, 449
Gigy, L. 198
Gilbert, B. 070
Gilligan, C. 458
Giummo, J. 557
Globus, Y. 558
Golan, M. 558
Golan, N. 473
Goldberg, E. 243
Goldberg, G. 037
Goldberg, S. 282
Goldstein, M. 452
Golub, S. 223
Gomez, E. 354
Gordon, E. 184
Grad, S. 135
Grambs, J. 490
Graney, M. 234
Greenaway, K. 099
Greene, V. 363
Gribbin, K. 232
Gropp, M. 496
Gross, Z. 011
Grow, J. 167
Grunebaum, H. 008
Guttman, D. 351, 362, 364, 368

H

Haddock, C. 043
Haga, H. 453
Hagestad, G. 038, 039
Hammer, B. 564
Hand, J. 037
Harel, Z. 328

Hartwigsen, G. 327
Hatfield, E. 065
Haug, M. 224, 325
Hawkins, J. 227
Hawkins, J. D. 332
Hayes, C. 351, 362, 364, 368
Hemmings, S. 499
Henig, R. 225
Henretta, J. 057, 126
Hepworth, M. 474
Hess, B. 041, 042, 122, 425
Higgins, C. 202
Hill, J. 566
Hing, E. 268
Hinrichsen, G. 329
Hirschfield, I. 500
Hochschild, A. 330
Hoffman, C. 164
Holahan, C. 530
Hollenshead, C. 501
Holloway, K. 365
Holt, N. 567
Homan, S. 043
Hooyman, N. 044
Horwitz, L. 597
Hottenstein, E. 100
Houser, R. 026
Hubley, F. 568
Hunn, D. 344
Hunsberger, B. 317
Hunt, H. 155
Hupp, S. 283

I

Iams, H. 136, 168
Ikels, C. 440
Ingersoll, B. 501
Irvin, Y. 410

J

Jackson, D. 532
Jackson, J. 357
Jackson, M. 328
Jacobs, R. 502
Jeffrey, B. 170
Jewson, R. 199
Johnsen, P. 028, 029, 164
Johnson, C. 045, 352
Johnson, C. K. 204
Johnson, E. S. 366
Johnson, S. 284

K

Kadom, W. 464
Kahne, H. 123, 169
Kalish, R. 351,
362, 364, 368
Kannel, W. 235
Kantrow, R. 037
Kaplan, B. 185
Katz, C. 501
Kaye, A. 101
Kaye, L. 200
Keating, N. 170
Keith, P. 201
Kennedy, C. 285
Kerns, V. 469
Kerzner, L. 236
Kiefer, C. 367
Kim, B.-L. 367
Kim, L. 367
Kim, S. 367
Kim, T. 367
King, N. 421
Kivett, V. 061, 318
Kleban, M. 164
Klein, L. 503
Klein, M. 239
Klodawsky, H. 132
Knight, C. 388
Koehler, B. 524
Koh, Y. 411
Kohen, J. 046
Koo, J. 465
Kopac, C. 286
Koyano, W. 453
Krach, M. 102
Kradlak, C. 209
Krause, N. 237
Kremen, E. 037
Kreps, J. 156
Kubelka, S. 475
Kungle, M. 255
Kunigonis, M. 221

L

LaCayo, C. 331
LaFont, P. 103
LaGory, M. 538
Lake, A. 226
Lalive d'Espinay, C. 454
Lally, M. 332
Lambert, T. 500
Landerman, R. 127
Landsberg, S. 010
Lang, A. 029
Langford, J. 287
Lasser, S. 288
Lauter, L. 037

Lee, C-F. 368
Lee, G. 205
Lesnoff-Caravaglia, G.
455, 504
Lesser, M. 289
Lev, Y. 524
Leverington, S. 577
Levy, S. 238
Lewis, M. 456
Lewis, V. 412
Liang, J. 369, 531
Lieberman D. 104
Lieberman, M. 358
Lipman, A. 048
Liss, B. 212
Litwin-Grinberg, R. 413
Logue, J. 241
Lohmann, N. 495
Lohr, M. 239
Long, J. 573
Long, J. 047
Longino, C. 048
Lopata, H. 012, 049, 050
Louie, D. 290
Luggen, A. 291
Luria, Z. 303

M

Macdonald, B. 014
Mackeracher, D. 619
Maddox, G. 038, 039,
041, 049, 052, 053,
055, 056, 122, 196,
248, 304, 331, 426,
505, 529, 536, 537
Madigan, M. 213
Manton, K. 370
Manuel, R. 353, 370,
371, 381, 446, 455
Manzella, D. 292
Mapz, B. 438
Margraff, R. 319
Markey, J. 476
Markides, K. 051,
354, 369, 372, 373
Markson, E. 027,
040, 042, 052, 173,
207, 229, 235, 236,
240, 306, 426, 506
Marshall, R. 157
Martin, C. 315, 316,
330, 332, 498
Martin, H. 354
Martineau, B. 336
Marton, D. 390
Marvel, M. 421
Massey, V. 105
Matthews, S. 013

Matsuzaki, T. 453
Maxwell, S. 186
Mazess, R. 457
McAuley, W. 333
McCallum, E. 257
McCrory, A. 106
McGannon, J. 391
McGloshen, T. 293
McIntosh, J. 242
McIlvaine, B. 507
McLaughlin, W. 294
McNeely, R. 355, 361, 374
Meacham, J. 528
Meade, R. 303
Melamed, E. 508
Melick, M. 241
Mellinger, J. 031
Mellstrom, D. 444
Meske, R. 310
Meyer, S. 414
Miller, E. 345
Miller, F. 575
Miller, J. 375
Miller, L. 511
Millette, B. 227
Mintz, J. 221
Moffett, M. 195
Mokin, A. 576
Monahan, D. 363
Monk, A. 200
Montgomery, R. 053
Moore, E. 487
Moore, J. 217
Morgan, L. 124, 125, 171
Moss, W. 107
Mouris, C. 577
Mundkur, M. 507
Murphy, J. 458
Murphy, M. 590
Murphy, S. 313

N

Nagy, M. 295
Nakazato, K. 453
Newman, E. 202
Noelker, L. 328
Norman, D. 458
Nudel, A. 228
Nunez, V. 393
Nusberg, C. 441
Nussbaum, A. 191

O

Obear, M. 296
Obomsawin, A. 395
O'Bryant, S. 054

O'Connell, P. 581
Oestreich, M. 187
Offerle, J. 333
Oliva, M. 259
O'Rand, A. 055, 056, 057, 126, 127
Ore, D. 583
Ory, M. 243
Owens, J. 076

P

Painter, C. 513
Palmore, E. 197, 316
Pampel, F. 459
Park, S. 459
Parsons, J. 396
Patrick, S. 397
Peabody, P. 077
Peace, S. 442
Pearlman, J. 007
Pearson, R. 448
Pellegrino, V. 477
Persson, G. 444
Peterson, N. 514
Phillips, G. 415
Pickering, M. 587
Pinsker, S. 078
Pimot, K. 620
Porcino, J. 515
Porter, K. 047, 147
Porter, N. 588
Post, L. 462
Powers, M. 416
Premo, T. 058, 621
Prentis, R. 203
Price-Bonham, S. 204
Primas, M. 148
Prince, N. 589
Puglisi, J. 532

R

Rabin, L. 488
Ralston, P. 376
Rao, V. N. 377
Rao, V. V. 377
Ray, L. 373
Raybeck, D. 443
Reid, J. 371
Replogle, M. 108
Rhodes, L. 590
Rich, C. 014
Rich-McCoy, L. 516
Riddick, C. 172
Ridley, J. 244
Rikli, R. 245
Rivers, C. 002
Rix, S. 121

Roberto, K. 059
Robertson, T. 260
Robbins, D. 008
Rodriguez, L. 051
Roebuck, J. 060
Rogers, N. 478
Rosen, A. 188
Rosen, E. 173
Rosenberger, N. 466
Roser, D. 221
Rosow, E. 462
Ross, J. 452
Rossi, A. 517
Rothblum, E. 222
Rotman, A. 214
Rubbo, M. 261
Rudnick, C. 606
Ryff, C. 032

S

Saalwaechter, K. 297
Sahara, P. 518
Sanchez-Ayendez, M. 417
Salmon, M. 129
Sanders, G. 109
Sands, J. 533
Sangster, E. 189
Santos, J. 242
Schabad, P.
Schaie, K. 232
Scharlach, A. 111
Schofield, R. 149
Schoonover, C. 164
Schreter, C. 346
Schuchardt, J. 150
Schuler, S. 452
Scott-Maxwell, F. 015
Scott, J. 059, 061
Sedney, M. 062
Seecombe, K. 205
Segalla, R. 016
Segedin, L. 497
Seskin, J. 017, 519, 520
Shabad, P. 110
Shands, A. 593
Sharma, M. 334
Shaw, D. 349
Shaw, L. 159, 160, 161, 206
Sheafor, M. 224
Sheehan, S. 018
Sherman, S. 202, 538
Shibata, H. 453
Shirley, R. 595
Shmueli, A. 450
Shon, S. 367
Shulman, A. 036
Silver, M. 151

Silverman, P. 019
Simmons, P. 521
Simon, J. 596
Sinnott, J. 246
Sky, L. 132
Sloan, B. 020
Smith, D. 314
Smith, L. 597
Snyder, P. 378
Sokolovsky, J. 441
Soldo, B. 334
Sommers, T. 298, 522
Spurlock, J. 379
Starr, B. 304
Steitz, J. 534
Sternberg, M. 467
Sternberg, T. 399
Stewart, P. 079
Stimson, A. 305
Stimson, J. 305
Stoddard, K. 523
Stone, A. 121
Stone, R. 269
Storandt, M. 230
Story, B. 347
Strate, J. 137
Strugnell, C. 021
Stuart, M. 080
Stueve, C. 112
Suyama, Y. 453
Svanborg, A. 444
Szinovacz, M. 126, 163, 166, 192, 199, 202, 204, 207, 423

T

Tai, V. 399
Tan, H. 599
Tate, L. 535
Taylor, R. 320, 357, 380, 418
Taylor, R. 600
Taylor, S. P. 381
Terry, R. 419
Teuter, U. 622
Thomas, J. 063
Thornock, M. 332
Thurnher, M. 064
Togonu-Bickersteth, F.460
Tracy, M. 128, 461
Traupmann, J. 065
Turner, B. 306, 536, 537
Tyer, Z. 031

U

Uhlenberg, P. 129

Usui, W. 382

V

Valois, P. 513
Vanden, J. 604
Van Tran, T. 369
Vasdudev, J. 458
Verbrugge, L. 247,248
Vernon, S. 372

W

Waciega, L. 113
Walker, G. 261
Walters, J. 114
Wambach, J. 115
Wang, W. 399
Ward, A. 383
Ward, R. L. 128
Ward, R. A. 538
Waring, J. 042
Warlick, J. 130
Wase, J. 305
Wasserman, P. 524
Wax, J. 479
Weaver, D. 299
Weiler, N. 436
Weinstein, E. 311
Welshufer, J. 255
Wengraf, S. 606
Wentowski, G. 066
Wershba, J. 177
Westoff, L. 480
Wharton, G. 301
Wheelwright, J. 525
Whisler, E. 116
Whitfield, P. 190
Whitted, M. 117
Wilson, K. 118
Winner, C. 043
Winogrond, I. 539
Wolf, J. 383
Wolinsky, F. 043
Wood, D. 481
Wu, S-C. 384
Wyckoff, S. 348

Y

Yeck, M. 322
Yu, L. 384
Yung, D. 399

Z

Zanuck, L. 610
Zanuck, R. 610
Ziegler, H. 3

About the Compiler

Jean M. Coyle, Ph.D., has been a social gerontologist for over a decade. She has published in the areas of entrepreneurial gerontology, women and retirement, and the rural black elderly.

Dr. Coyle is President of Jean Coyle Associates, a gerontological consulting firm based in Alexandria, Virginia. Dr. Coyle directs The National Institute of Senior Centers and The National Association of Older Worker Employment Services, affiliate units of The National Council on the Aging, Inc., in Washington, D.C.

Dr. Coyle founded the first academic gerontology program in the state of Louisiana in 1976. She also has taught at universities in Indiana, Texas, Illinois, Washington, D.C., and Virginia, and held a tenured associate professorship.

Jean Coyle is Founding President of The International Association of Gerontological Entrepreneurs, serves on the boards of a number of gerontological and business organizations, and has held office in various professional groups at national, regional, and state levels.

The author holds B.A., M.A., and Ph.D. degrees in sociology. She has completed study in gerontology at the University of Michigan and in business management at the University of Virginia.